SpringerBriefs in Public Health

SpringerBriefs in Public Health present concise summaries of cutting-edge research and practical applications from across the entire field of public health, with contributions from medicine, bioethics, health economics, public policy, biostatistics, and sociology.

The focus of the series is to highlight current topics in public health of interest to a global audience, including health care policy; social determinants of health; health issues in developing countries; new research methods; chronic and infectious disease epidemics; and innovative health interventions.

Featuring compact volumes of 50 to 125 pages, the series covers a range of content from professional to academic. Possible volumes in the series may consist of timely reports of state-of-the art analytical techniques, reports from the field, snapshots of hot and/or emerging topics, elaborated theses, literature reviews, and in-depth case studies. Both solicited and unsolicited manuscripts are considered for publication in this series.

Briefs are published as part of Springer's eBook collection, with millions of users worldwide. In addition, Briefs are available for individual print and electronic purchase.

Briefs are characterized by fast, global electronic dissemination, standard publishing contracts, easy-to-use manuscript preparation and formatting guidelines, and expedited production schedules. We aim for publication 8–12 weeks after acceptance.

More information about this series at http://www.springer.com/series/10138

Saroj Pachauri · Ash Pachauri ·
Komal Mittal

Sexual and Reproductive Health and Rights in India

Self-care for Universal Health Coverage

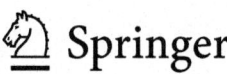

Saroj Pachauri
New Delhi, India

Ash Pachauri
Center for Human Progress
New Delhi, India

Komal Mittal
Center for Human Progress
New Delhi, India

ISSN 2192-3698 ISSN 2192-3701 (electronic)
SpringerBriefs in Public Health
ISBN 978-981-16-4577-8 ISBN 978-981-16-4578-5 (eBook)
https://doi.org/10.1007/978-981-16-4578-5

© The Author(s) 2022. This book is an open access publication.
Open Access This book is licensed under the terms of the Creative Commons Attribution 4.0 International License (http://creativecommons.org/licenses/by/4.0/), which permits use, sharing, adaptation, distribution and reproduction in any medium or format, as long as you give appropriate credit to the original author(s) and the source, provide a link to the Creative Commons license and indicate if changes were made.

The images or other third party material in this book are included in the book's Creative Commons license, unless indicated otherwise in a credit line to the material. If material is not included in the book's Creative Commons license and your intended use is not permitted by statutory regulation or exceeds the permitted use, you will need to obtain permission directly from the copyright holder.

The use of general descriptive names, registered names, trademarks, service marks, etc. in this publication does not imply, even in the absence of a specific statement, that such names are exempt from the relevant protective laws and regulations and therefore free for general use.

The publisher, the authors and the editors are safe to assume that the advice and information in this book are believed to be true and accurate at the date of publication. Neither the publisher nor the authors or the editors give a warranty, expressed or implied, with respect to the material contained herein or for any errors or omissions that may have been made. The publisher remains neutral with regard to jurisdictional claims in published maps and institutional affiliations.

This Springer imprint is published by the registered company Springer Nature Singapore Pte Ltd.
The registered company address is: 152 Beach Road, #21-01/04 Gateway East, Singapore 189721, Singapore

Foreword

This book is a very important addition to the extensive range of research and writing that Dr. Saroj Pachauri has contributed to the knowledge and intervention strategies concerning health issues in India and Asia. The book focuses on developing greater depths of scientific data and new programmatic strategies for sexual and reproductive health in especially marginalized, vulnerable sub-groups—female sex workers, men who have sex with men (MSM), transgender people, and long distance truck drivers.

As evident in the title of the book, the primary theme is the up-scaling of self-care practices, particularly among the most vulnerable sub-populations in India. Dr. Pachauri states: "The COVID-19 pandemic currently raging through India and other countries vividly underscores the importance of self-care interventions. All the methods to prevent this infection such as hand washing, social/physical distancing, and wearing masks are self-care interventions. Without a vaccine to prevent this infection, individuals and communities are reliant solely on self-care practices."

These most vulnerable sub-groups are especially at risk because of their exposure to a variety of different, unpredictable sexual encounters, and also their relatively weak and unstable economic and social resources. In addition, these sub-groups generally have low levels of knowledge concerning the pathways and risks of sexually transmitted infections and related health problems, along with (frequently) a serious lack of connections to reliable, effective health providers.

The first "vulnerable subpopulation" for which data are presented from recent research is the category, "men who have sex with men" (MSM) in Chap. 2. Dr. Pachauri and colleagues quickly point out that, especially in India, that label MSM includes a very wide range of different kinds of individuals, with widely different sexual activities and varied levels of knowledge of health risks and resources. Research in India needs to explore in more depth the practices and perceptions of the important categories. As noted in Chap. 2, "In India the term MSM encompasses many identities, gender constructs, and communities. It includes a wide range of distinct categories of men who self-identify themselves as gay, bisexual, transgender or heterosexual and engage in sex with other men".

That situation leads to this important statement: "There is a critical need to understand and integrate identities and self-concepts that inform sexual behavior. Inclusive discussions on sexual identity that recognize diversity of ideas in sexual behavior are critical because male sexual behaviors have been inadequately constructed".

Chapter 3 presents data concerning transgender persons, which in India are mainly people previously referred to as hijras in most regions, but with various other labels as well. Most of the transgender individuals were born as males, but developed strong feminine characteristics while growing to adulthood. "An older name for hijras is kinnar, which is used by some hijra groups as a more respectable and formal term".

As in practically all aspects of socio-cultural structures in India, there are significant differences in the situations of hijras in different states and regions. Dr. Pachauri and colleagues point out that in the state of Tamil Nadu these transgender individuals and groups, are termed aravanis, and have better societal and legal status than in other states. In 2008 the state government established the Tamil Nadu Aravanigal Welfare Board, under the Department of Social Welfare. The Aravanigal Board has initiated systems of income assistance, housing, employment, health care, and other programs for improving living conditions of the aravani communities.

Unlike most other marginalized, socially abused persons in India, the "real hijras" generally live in groups ("families"), in which there is one individual who is the guru (mentor, and also identified as "mother"). In addition, some individuals are gurus for a wider network of hijras, particularly in urban areas. In some locations (e.g., Mumbai) hijras stated that they hand over all their earnings to their guru, who in turn, gives out money as needed by various "family members." Some aravanis in Tamil Nadu, however, reported that they don't turn over their earnings to their guru, but they generally give gifts to the guru on various occasions. The general hijra/aravani pattern of living in "family groups" suggests that programs focused on developing stronger self-care concepts and actions can be built around those "family structures."

Based on the current state of data about transgender persons and groups in India, the researchers stated: "Self-care among transgender has an important place in improving their health and their lives. Self-care is practiced by many transgender but there is considerable scope for improvement. Research is needed to assess how and in which areas self-care can be enhanced to improve the lives of transgender. Growing access to the internet has facilitated the process of increasing self- care to improve the health and well-being of transgender."

In the chapter on female sex workers (FSWs), Dr. Pachauri and her colleagues note that considerable progress has been made in improved health care and self-care practices in this very large sub-population. Those developments resulted from the intensive community-based programs for countering the spread of HIV/AIDS during the past three decades. However, more research and action programs are needed because of the complex, highly varied categories of FSWs. As pointed out in the extensive research literature, there are large differences in the situations of brothel-based, street-based and home-based sex workers. In addition, quite different situations of sex-work, health care, and support systems are found among the devadasis who are the majority of sex workers in northern Karnataka and some other locations. The researchers pointed out that "Migrant sex workers are particularly at high risk of HIV". Very little research has focused on the migrant FSWs. Of course there are other sub-categories of sex workers, in addition to which, regional variations and rural-versus-urban contexts add to the complexities that need further careful study.

The internationally well-known Sonagachi Program in Kolkata is a particularly central case example for development of comprehensive self-care programs. Pachauri and associates wrote: "The Sonagachi Project in Kolkata, West Bengal, Durbar is the longest running empowerment-based HIV prevention program for female sex workers in India, serving more than 65,000 female sex workers annually". The Sonagachi program (Initiated in 1992) has had multiple research episodes, and serves as a model for further, more advanced studies, in other programs and regions. This chapter concerning female sex workers is particularly valuable because of the extensive mass of references. A total of 85 publications are listed.

The long distance truckers are a distinctly different kind of vulnerable sub-population. "India has a large trucking population… and about 2–2.5 million are classified as long distance truckers". A major factor inducing greater vulnerability in the long distance trucking population is that they are very frequently away from their homes and families for long periods. "A study by Chaturvedi et al., in 2006, showed that truck drivers who were away from home for more than 20 days were 15 times more likely to have exposure to female sex workers".

In addition to the frequent occurrence of long "on the road" situations, several of the studies reviewed by Pachauri and her colleagues indicated a variety of difficulties and harassments endured by the truckers. A very interesting case history of a 28-year-old trucker from Haryana quotes him as saying that he never should have taken up this occupation. Concerning harassment by the police, he described: "On the Rajasthan-Jaipur road, there are so many RTOs (Regional Transport Officers) who check my truck, and even when it is not overloaded, they take money from me like 500–1000 rupees. If I do not give them the money, they beat me," says Sahabudin. This informant also talked about problems with thieves and other trouble-makers.

The case histories in this chapter greatly enhance descriptions about the complexities in the daily experiences of the truck drivers and their helpers ("cleaners"). Further complications include the apparently high rates of alcohol consumption in at least some sectors of the trucker population. Some studies reported in the chapter found strong correlations of alcohol use and going to female sex workers.

In the way forward (chapter 6), Dr. Pachauri and her co-authors state that, "The field of self-care interventions is new, fast moving, and multi-disciplinary. There is a need to explore the way ahead in advancing the field so that self-care forms an integral part of health programs. In order to move this agenda forward, a comprehensive strategy is needed."

The first major point in the conclusions focuses on significant changes in the training of health professionals. "New approaches in training and education of healthcare providers are needed in order to institutionalize sensitive and effective use of self-care interventions. Health care providers include doctors, nurses, midwives, community health workers and pharmacists among others."

Another major theme in the conclusions focuses on the "self-care technologies." Those include a variety of materials, ranging from oral contraceptives (and various other means of contraception) to self-testing equipment and effective means of instruction for their use, pre- and post-exposure prophylaxis, and various other old and new self-care materials.

Of course, the education of potential users in marginalized, vulnerable populations requires careful attention and organization. Some of that can be incorporated in mass media. The evidence from the various HIV/AIDS programs in India points to the central importance of various community-based organizations, including FSW collectives and their outreach workers, in person-to-person educational activities regarding effective use of self-care technologies. With regard to accessing self-care technology and effective information, Dr. Pachauri and colleagues noted that, "Mobile apps and online ordering services have become new intermediaries with internet drug stores and pharmacies".

While much of the research and development of programmatic actions is focused on the marginalized communities, there is also a need to develop more effective advocacy for reaching policy-makers at various governmental levels. The concluding chapter points out that, "Strong policy advocacy made it possible to acknowledge the legal rights of transgender. Policy advocacy undertaken jointly by NGOs, lawyers, researchers and the community itself, made it possible to convince policy-makers to recognize their special needs and to frame appropriate laws for the transgender community".

As pointed out at the beginning of this writing, the main purpose of the book is to present a framework for advancement of "self-care as an integral part of health programs and individual rights" among the vulnerable populations. The descriptions of the special target populations, and the extensive lists of references make up that frame of reference. For programmatic developments in each of those sub-populations, effective, in-depth research is needed. Dr. Pachauri places strong emphasis on qualitative research methods as highly effective ways to get the kinds of detailed information needed for program development in specific community sub-groups.

Dr. Pertti J. Pelto
Former Chair
Department of Cultural Anthropology
University of Connecticut
Mansfield, CT, USA

Preface

Self-care is a new, fast-moving, multidisciplinary field. People have been practicing self-care for millennia but new products, information and technologies are changing how health services are delivered. Self-care compliments healthcare systems to achieve the goal of universal health coverage (UHC). UHC is a people-centered approach that views people as important decision-makers who can take charge of their own health with evidence-based self-care interventions.

In this volume, the rationale and concept for self-care are discussed. The framework for self-care for a comprehensive approach to sexual and reproductive health and rights focusing on the most marginalized and vulnerable populations is also examined.

Four case studies are presented. These case studies include the results of qualitative research undertaken in different states of India on men who have sex with men (MSM), transgender, female sex workers (FSWs) and long distance truck drivers. Research questions address their perceptions and experiences, their motivations for using self-care, the barriers they face, and the mechanisms they employ when self-care fails. Personal narratives of community members provide deep insights into their lived experience. Workshops provided a platform to these communities for sharing their perceptions, experiences, difficulties encountered, and motivations for using self-care services and products. Artwork by the community members pictorially illustrates their perceptions and experiences with self-care. These novel, creative and innovative methodologies enabled the researchers to study these hard-to-reach communities.

Training of health professionals, education of the community, availability and accessibility of self- care technologies, digital and online resources to accelerate self-care and research-based evidence to formulate policies and programs for moving the agenda forward are discussed. And key questions for future research driven by a collaborative ethos are also delienated.

New Delhi, India
Saroj Pachauri
Ash Pachauri
Komal Mittal

Acknowledgements

I am deeply grateful to the World Health Organization (WHO) for the generous support provided for undertaking workshops with vulnerable and marginalized communities. The artwork presented throughout the publication was generated by these communities as an outcome from the WHO-supported workshops. The result of these workshops complemented the research which provides the basis for the discussions for self-care in this volume.

It was the encouragement, inspiration and support of my family that helped me to complete this volume through difficult times. My husband Patchy, inspired and cajoled me to begin writing. Constant encouragement by my daughters Rashmi and Shonali and my dear friend and sister Dr. Anjali Saha kept me going. Rashmi and Philo Magdalene wrote personal narratives of the community members which have added great value to the research by providing insights into their lived experiences. Rashmi also assisted with the field research.

I thank Mr. Manish Gupta for his assistance in many administrative chores that were required throughout the process of writing this volume. He also assisted with the field research and workshops.

Dr. Ash Pachauri, my co-author inspired me throughout the process. Discussions with him were invaluable. He also organized and moderated the workshops. Ms. Komal Mittal also accompanied us on this journey as a co-author. I thank her for undertaking the analysis of the research findings and assisting with the field research. As partners on this journey, we encountered moments of great joy and fulfillment and also went through many arguments and disagreements.

This volume is based on a subject which is as yet nascent and, therefore, very challenging. It is the outcome of the unwavering support and encouragement of my family and friends to whom I owe a deep sense of gratitude.

Contents

1 **Self-care: Concept, Rationale, and Framework** 1
   1.1 Concept and Rationale for Self-care....................... 1
   1.2 Framework for Self-care 2
   1.3 WHO Guideline on Sexual and Reproductive Health
       and Rights 4
   1.4 Sole Reliance on Self-care for Preventing COVID-19 5
   1.5 Innovative Research Methodology 5
   References 6

2 **Men Who Have Sex with Men** 9
   2.1 Backdrop... 9
   2.2 Research on MSM 10
   2.3 Research Findings 11
       2.3.1 An Expression of the Feelings and Behaviors
            of MSM 11
       2.3.2 Self-care Interventions for Sexual and Reproductive
            Health 12
       2.3.3 Information Sources for Sexual and Reproductive
            Health 13
       2.3.4 Risks and Barriers Faced by the Community 15
       2.3.5 Mental Health Issues Faced by the Community 16
       2.3.6 Violence Faced by the Community 17
       2.3.7 Motivation for Self-care 17
   2.4 From Vulnerability to Resilience 18
       2.4.1 MSM's Personal Narrative on Self-care.............. 18
   2.5 Discussion 22
   References 24

3 **Understanding Health Needs of Transgender** 27
   3.1 Backdrop... 27

	3.2	Research on Transgender	28
		3.2.1 Research Findings	29
		3.2.2 Reflections of Transgender	29
		3.2.3 Self-care Interventions for Sexual and Reproductive Health	30
		3.2.4 Information Sources for Sexual and Reproductive Health	31
		3.2.5 Risks and Barriers Faced by the Community	32
		3.2.6 Violence Faced by the Community	33
		3.2.7 Mental Health Issues Faced by the Community	35
		3.2.8 Motivations for Self-care	35
		3.2.9 A Transgender's Personal Narrative on Self-care	35
	3.3	Discussion	39
	References		41
4	**Female Sex Work Dynamics: Empowerment, Mobilization, Mobility**		**43**
	4.1	Backdrop	43
	4.2	Research on Female Sex Workers	44
		4.2.1 Research Findings	45
		4.2.2 Involvement in Sex Work	45
		4.2.3 Self-care Interventions for Health and Family Planning	46
		4.2.4 Information Sources	47
		4.2.5 Risks and Barriers Faced by the Community	48
		4.2.6 Mental Health Problems Faced by the Community	48
		4.2.7 Violence Faced by the Community	48
		4.2.8 Motivation for Self-care	49
		4.2.9 A Female Sex Worker with AIDS: Personal Narrative on Self-care	50
	4.3	Discussion	53
	References		56
5	**Sexual Behaviors of Long-Distance Truck Drivers**		**61**
	5.1	Backdrop	61
	5.2	Research on Long-Distance Truck Drivers	62
		5.2.1 Research Findings	62
		5.2.2 Lifestyle of Long-Distance Truck Drivers	63
		5.2.3 Sexual Behaviors of Long-Distance Truck Drivers	64
		5.2.4 Self-care Interventions for Sexual and Reproductive Health	64
		5.2.5 Information Sources	65
		5.2.6 Issues Related to Cost and Affordability	66
		5.2.7 Risks and Barriers Faced by the Community	66

		5.2.8	Mental Health Problems and Violence	66
		5.2.9	Motivations for Self-care	67
		5.2.10	A Personal Narrative by a Member of the Trucking Community	67
		5.2.11	A Long-Distance Truck Driver's Personal Narrative on Self-care	69
	5.3	Discussion		71
	References			73
6	**The Way Forward**			77
	6.1	Training Health Professionals on SRHR Self-care Interventions		77
	6.2	Education of Potential Users on Self-care		78
	6.3	Self-care Technologies		79
	6.4	Digital and Online Resources on Self-care		79
	6.5	Research-Based Evidence for Policies and Programs		80
	References			82

About the Authors

Saroj Pachauri a Public Health Physician has undertaken extensive research on sexual and reproductive health and rights, HIV and AIDS, family planning, maternal health, gender, poverty and youth. Saroj Pachauri was Regional Director for South and East Asia, Population Council. She has published 4 books, contributed chapters to 20 books, published over 100 papers in peer-reviewed journals and numerous print and media articles. She was awarded the Grants Gold Medal for securing the first position in DPH and was bestowed the prestigious title of Distinguished Scholar by the Population Council.

Ash Pachauri a Ph.D. in Behavioral Science and a Public Health Expert, is a Self-Care Guideline Development Group Member of the World Health Organization, Geneva. He was awarded the exclusive Overseas Research Scholarship by the Secretary of State for Education and Science, UK; awarded a full scholarship for a Ford Foundation-funded Sexual Health Education Program by San Francisco State University; and honored with the "Portraits of Commitment" leadership title by the United Nations. He has contributed to five books and authored over 55 conference papers and publications.

Komal Mittal is Research Associate in health at the Center for Human Progress and is a Global Youth Mentor with the POP (Protect Our Planet) Movement. She has conducted research on understanding self-care practices of the most marginalized and vulnerable communities in India. Komal Mittal led a national youth group supported by UNAIDS which focused on promoting leadership and advocacy for the Sustainable Development Goals. She has attended several conferences, including some internationally, and has presented several reports on public health issues. She was awarded the "Research Excellence Award" in the field of biotechnology for a study on "Extraction of Acid Soluble Collagen from Soybean and Tomato".

Acronyms

ACA	Affordable Care Act
AIDS	Acquired Immunodeficiency Syndrome
ART	Antiretroviral Therapy
CBOs	Community-Based Organizations
CCU	Consistent Condom Use
FGDs	Focus Group Discussions
FGM	Female Genital Mutilation
FSWs	Female Sex Workers
HIV	Human Immunodeficiency Virus
HPV	Human Papillomavirus
HST	Humsafar Trust
IBBA	Integrated Behavioral and Biological Assessment
ICTCs	Integrated Counseling and Training Centers
IDIs	In-depth Interviews
KIIs	Key Informant Interviews
LGBTQ	Lesbian, Gay, Bisexual, Transgender and Queer
MSM	Men who have Sex with Men
NCHSR	National Center for Health Services Research
NFI	Naz Foundation International
NGOs	Non-Governmental Organizations
OOP	Out-Of-Pocket
PrEP	Pre-Exposure Prophylaxis
RTOs	Regional Transport Officers
S/UIIs	Self or User Initiated Interventions
SGTN	Sanjay Gandhi Transport Nagar
SRH	Sexual and Reproductive Health
SRHR	Sexual and Reproductive Health and Rights
SRS	Sex Reassignment Surgery
STIs	Sexually Transmitted Infections
TB	Tuberculosis

TGNC	Transgender and Gender Non-Confirming
UHC	Universal Health Coverage
UIDAI	Unique Identification Development Authority of India
UNAIDS	United Nations for Acquired Immunodeficiency Syndrome
UNDP	United Nations Development Programme
WHO	World Health Organization

Chapter 1
Self-care: Concept, Rationale, and Framework

1.1 Concept and Rationale for Self-care

The role and importance of self-care in the continuum of health care are becoming important subjects of debate among social scientists and health professionals. Interest in the self-care component of health services is stimulated by the convergence of diverse pressures common to health services systems. Depersonalized medical care, rising costs of high technology, focus on curative care, growth of lay knowledge, recognition of the limits of medical care and documentation of the impact of the individual's health behavior on patterns of morbidity are all factors stimulating new thinking regarding the importance of individuals and families to the effective and efficient functioning of health service systems.

The National Center for Health Services Research (NCHSR) organized the first national-level meeting in the USA on this topic in 1976. One of the conclusions was that baseline studies on the current extent of self-care practice were needed. The premise underlying the first international symposium on the role of the individual in primary health care held at the Institute of Social Medicine, University of Copenhagen, in 1975 was that a viable preventive and therapeutic partnership between individuals, patients and families, and professional healthcare workers is not only desirable, but may be essential to achieve improved access, enhanced quality of care, better accountability, and lower costs [1].

People have been practicing self-care for millennia, but new products, information, and technologies are changing how health services are delivered. The provider-to-receiver model that is at the heart of many health systems must be complemented with a self-care model through which people can be empowered to prevent, test for, and treat diseases themselves. A clear solution is to work toward universal health coverage (UHC), which not only improves health outcomes, but can help to reduce poverty, promote gender equality, and protect the most vulnerable populations. UHC is a people-centered approach that views people as active decision-makers in their own health and not merely passive recipients of health services. A people-centered approach supports health literacy so that people can take charge of their own health with evidence-based self-care interventions. When people have agency and autonomy, they can make and enact decisions in all aspects of their lives, including in relation to sexuality and reproduction.

Today, at least half the world's people have no access to essential health services, including 214 million women of reproductive age in developing countries who want methods to avoid pregnancy. An estimated 22 million unsafe abortions occur worldwide each year, more than one million sexually transmitted infections are acquired every day, and worldwide, the number of new HIV infections among young people is not declining [2].

1.2 Framework for Self-care

A comprehensive approach to sexual and reproductive health and rights (SRHR) covers maternal and perinatal health, family planning, infertility, abortion, sexually transmitted infections (STIs) including HIV, reproductive system cancers, gynecological morbidities, and sexual health, as well as several cross-cutting themes such as gender-based violence.

Within the framework of WHO's definition of health, as a state of complete physical, mental, and social well-being, and not merely the absence of disease or infirmity, sexual and reproductive health (SRH) addresses sexuality and sexual relationships as well as the reproductive processes, functions, and system at all stages of life. Ensuring the full implementation of human rights-based laws and policies through SRH programs is fundamental to health and rights. Implicit in this are a wide range of human rights relating to SRH including the rights of men and women to have pleasurable and safe sexual experiences free of coercion, discrimination and violence, the right to be informed of and have access to safe, effective, affordable, and acceptable methods of fertility regulation of their choice, and the right of access to appropriate health services that will enable women to go safely through pregnancy and childbirth and provide couples with the best chance of having a healthy infant.

Some examples include health promotion activities (e.g., voluntary family planning, self-testing for HIV other STIs or pregnancy, or seeking advice and information through mHealth); disease prevention and control activities (e.g., practicing safe sex when condoms are consistently and correctly used to prevent unintended pregnancy and STIs, including HIV); and self-treatment and medication (e.g., contraception, self-management of abortion by taking oral misoprostol, or self-administered antibiotics made available without prescription through pharmacies to treat STIs) [2].

The WHO Constitution states that: *"The enjoyment of the highest attainable standard of health is one of the fundamental rights of every human being without distinction of race, religion, political belief, economic or social condition"* [3]. In order to ensure that WHO normative guidelines support the realization of the right to health of all, it is fundamental to their development that equity, human rights, gender, and the social determinants of health are taken into consideration. In the case of self-care intervention it is, therefore, essential to place particular emphasis on the needs of populations who may neither be aware of their right to health nor be able to access the services they need. These include vulnerable, marginalized, and socio-economically underprivileged populations who have the poorest health outcomes globally.

Vulnerability depends on the context and can be experienced across diverse populations including, but not limited to, individuals who: are lesbian, gay, bisexual, transgender, or intersex; use or have used drugs; are or have been involved in sex work; are separated, divorced or widowed; have undergone female genital mutilation (FGM); are living with HIV, tuberculosis (TB), malaria, hepatitis B or C, and/or other infections; are currently or have previously been incarcerated, detained or homeless; are economic or political migrants; are living with disabilities, including learning disabilities; are from minority ethnic groups; are elderly with reduced intrinsic capacity and/or are adolescents.

The World Health Organization's working definition of self-care includes "*the ability of individuals, families and, communities to promote health, prevent disease, maintain health, and cope with illness and disability with or without the support of a health-care provider.*" While this is a broad definition that includes many activities, it is important for self-care, especially where it intersects with health systems and health professionals. The recent global conference on primary health care, which celebrated the 40th anniversary of the Alma Ata declaration, again underscored the importance of empowering and supporting people in acquiring the knowledge, skills, and resources needed to maintain their health or the health of those for whom they care [4].

In recent years, the market for drugs, devices, and diagnostics has significantly increased globally. Digital technologies have also increased rapidly and are continuing to do so. This is resulting in new configurations of self-care. The impact of these changes on programs and policies needs to be understood.

Individuals choose a self-care health intervention for many positive reasons including convenience, cost, empowerment, and a better fit with values or lifestyle. A proven efficacy and endorsement by the health system may be another reason to choose self-care interventions. Given that an ideal, well-functioning health system is seldom a reality, particularly in resource-constrained settings, individuals may also opt for self-care interventions to avoid the health system owing to poor quality services or because information, interventions, or products are inappropriate, unaffordable, or inaccessible. Stigma from healthcare providers or from within families and communities may be another reason people turn to self-care. Self-care interventions fulfill a particularly important role in these situations, as the alternative might be no access at all to health promoting interventions [5].

The conceptual framework for self-care acknowledges that while there are traditional self-care practices, people are accessing new information and products through a variety of channels including pharmacies and the Internet. There is a phenomenal increase in mobile technologies and digital health for self-care. An enabling policy and legal environment that is supportive and safe is also essential for the implementation of safe and high-quality self-care interventions [6].

Some self-care interventions such as condoms are fully controlled by the individual. Others require interaction with the health service system. For example, HIV self-testing requires confirmation by the health system. Others such as HPV self-testing require the health system to do the test. Thus, the support of the health system is needed for implementing some self-care interventions.

Self-care is especially important for vulnerable populations because they are unable to access the health service system primarily because they are stigmatized by healthcare providers. This is especially true in the case of services for sexual and reproductive health and rights because vulnerable populations do not have the autonomy over their bodies to make decisions about sexuality and reproduction.

1.3 WHO Guideline on Sexual and Reproductive Health and Rights

In 2019, WHO issued a guideline on sexual and reproductive health self-care interventions. The guideline addresses a wide range of issues including antenatal care, childbirth, postpartum and newborn care, family planning, safe abortion, STIs including HIV, and sexual health. The purpose of the guideline is to provide people-centered, evidence-based guidance to individuals, communities, and countries to promote quality health services and self-care interventions based on public health strategies. Evidence-based self-care recommended by WHO includes information on sexual and reproductive health issues as well as on ways in which individuals can obtain drugs and devices. Many diagnostics and digital products can be used with or without the direct supervision of a health provider. Some examples are self-injectable contraceptives, self-sampling kits, and HIV self-tests [4].

Ensuring an enabling environment in which self-care interventions can be made available in safe, and appropriate ways must be a key initial piece of any strategy to introduce or scale-up these interventions. This should be informed by the profile of potential users, the services on offer to them, the broader legal and policy environment, and structural support and barriers [4].

Marginalized and vulnerable communities including lesbian, gay, bisexual, and transgender (LGBT) communities, truck drivers, female sex workers, HIV positive people, among others, have social, economic, and political problems which result in health consequences. These communities suffer from stigma and discrimination. Because of their economic conditions and cultural beliefs, they have little access to formal healthcare services. Their basic human rights are violated, and they face discrimination in society as well as in the health system. For example, people with same-sex preferences are ridiculed and ostracized by their families and also by society. While health programs may achieve their goals by improving the well-being of easy-to-reach communities, they may exacerbate inequality if hard-to-reach populations are left behind. There is ample evidence to show that LGBT communities are hard-to-reach [7–9]. Therefore, it is important to undertake research to capture their self-care practices, values, and preferences, especially with regard to SRHR and HIV prevention.

In line with the WHO conceptual framework for self-care interventions, there are two complimentary pathways of change to improve health and well-being: increasing autonomy and agency through empowering individuals, particularly vulnerable populations, to advance SRHR; and transforming the health system approach to create a safe and supportive enabling environment to serve vulnerable populations. In line with the process of the development of WHO global normative guidance on self-care interventions, continued engagement of healthcare providers as well as the self-careers and care-givers has the potential to transform *ad hoc* activities into policies and programs for implementation that improves SRH, human rights, and UHC [10].

1.4 Sole Reliance on Self-care for Preventing COVID-19

The COVID-19 pandemic currently raging through India and several other countries vividly underscores the importance of self-care interventions. All the methods to prevent this infection such as hand washing, social/physical distancing, and wearing masks are self-care interventions. Without a vaccine to prevent this infection, individuals and communities are reliant solely on self-care practices. The COVID-19 pandemic has made both healthcare practitioners and users of health services cognizant of the critical need for promoting and scaling-up self-care interventions. Serious efforts are underway globally to achieve this goal. WHO has developed a communication media tool kit and a social media kit for sexual and reproductive health and COVID-19 [11].

The problem of waste management of self-care products needs redressal [12]. Significantly exacerbated by the COVID-19 pandemic, the problem of waste management needs to be better understood so that effective and sustainable strategies can be implemented to manage the uncontrolled growth of self-care waste.

1.5 Innovative Research Methodology

In this volume, four case studies are presented. These case studies include the results of research undertaken on vulnerable and marginalized communities in several different states of the country. Qualitative research was undertaken on men who have sex with men (MSM), transgender, female sex workers (FSWs), and long-distance truck drivers. Research questions addressed their perceptions and experience with self-care, their sources of information, their motivations for using self-care, the barriers they encountered, and the mechanisms they employed when self-care failed.

Quotes are generously used to amplify the voices of the members of these marginalized and vulnerable communities. Research results are supplemented with literature reviews. In addition, personal narratives of community members provide invaluable insights into their lived experience.

The case studies discuss the evolution of self-care interventions and their impact on the health of the community, in particular on sexual and reproductive health and HIV prevention. These also include a discussion of reproductive rights which are seriously violated in these communities. Issues related to stigma and discrimination and violence among these communities are highlighted. And finally, factors that resulted in changes in policies and programs to improve their sexual and reproductive health and grant them the right to health, education and employment are discussed. The case studies provide an understanding of what worked and what did not in mobilizing and empowering these vulnerable communities.

In addition to the research, a number of workshops were organized in several states of India to provide a platform for discussion for these communities. At these workshops, the community members expressed their perceptions of self-care interventions and their experience in using them. They also shared the difficulties and obstacles that they faced and their motivations for using self-care services and products. Artwork by the community members illustrated the communities' need for and experience with self-care. Research ethics and confidentiality were strictly adhered to during the research. Thus, novel, creative, and innovative methodologies were employed to study these hard-to-reach communities.

In the following four chapters, the case studies on MSM, transgender, FSWs, and long-distance truck drivers are presented. The last chapter examines how the agenda on self-care can be advanced in the years ahead.

The audience for this publication includes health professionals, those managing health institutions and service providers. Researchers, donors, and professionals in the field of information technology would also find these writings of value in their work. Since this volume discusses a subject that is of interest to the general public and is written in an easy-to-read style, it would attract broader audiences, especially potential users of self-care interventions.

References

1. Dean K. Self-care responses to illness: A selected review. Soc Sci Med. 1981;1(15A):673–87.
2. World Health Organization. Preventing unsafe abortion. Geneva: World Health Organization; 2019.
3. Narasimhan M, Allotey P, Hardon A. Self-care interventions to advance health and well-being: A conceptual framework to inform normative guidance. BMJ Suppl. 2019;1:3–6.
4. World Health Organization. WHO consolidated guideline on self-care interventions for health: Sexual and reproductive health and rights. Geneva: World Health Organization; 2019.

References

5. World Health Organization. Ethical, legal & human rights and social accountability of self-initiated interventions. Brocher Meeting Report. Geneva: World Health Organization; 2018.
6. World Health Organization. WHO guidelines for digital health interventions. Geneva: World Health Organization; 2016.
7. Bains S, Egede L. Associations between health literacy, diabetes knowledge, self-care behaviors, and glycemic control in a low-income population with type 2 diabetes. Diabetes Technol Ther. 2011;13(3):335–41.
8. Avis M, Bulman D, Leighton P. Factors affecting participation in 'Sure Start' Programmes: A qualitative investigation of parents' views. Health Soc Care Community. 2007;15(3):203–11.
9. Barlow J, Kirkpatrick S, Stewart-Brown S, Davis H. Hard-to-reach or out-of-reach? Reasons why women refuse to take part in early interventions. Child Soc. 2005;19:199–210.
10. Narasimhan M, Logie CH, Gauntley A, Ponce de Leon RG, Gholbzouri K, Siegfried N, Abela H, Ouedraogo L. Self-care interventions for sexual and reproductive health and rights for advancing universal health coverage. Sex Reprod Health Matters. https://doi.org/10.1080/26410397. 2020. 1778610.
11. World Health Organization. Self-care interventions for health: Sexual and reproductive health and rights. Communications tool kit. Geneva: World Health Organization; 2020.
12. Pachauri A, Shah P, Almroth BC, Sevilla NPM, Narasimhan M. Safe and sustainable management of self-care products. BMJ Suppl. 2019;1:20–3.

Open Access This chapter is licensed under the terms of the Creative Commons Attribution 4.0 International License (http://creativecommons.org/licenses/by/4.0/), which permits use, sharing, adaptation, distribution and reproduction in any medium or format, as long as you give appropriate credit to the original author(s) and the source, provide a link to the Creative Commons license and indicate if changes were made.

The images or other third party material in this chapter are included in the chapter's Creative Commons license, unless indicated otherwise in a credit line to the material. If material is not included in the chapter's Creative Commons license and your intended use is not permitted by statutory regulation or exceeds the permitted use, you will need to obtain permission directly from the copyright holder.

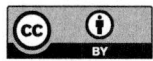

Chapter 2
Men Who Have Sex with Men

2.1 Backdrop

Men who have sex with men (MSM) are men who engage in sexual activity with members of the same sex, regardless of how they identify themselves. In India, same-sex behavior and relations tend to be much more fluid. These men may identify as gay, homosexual, bisexual, heterosexual, or may dispense with sexual identity altogether [1]. Indian terms are *kothi* (receptive or effeminate male partner), *panthi* (stereotypically penetrative or masculine male partner), "double deckers" (men who engage in both penetrative and receptive anal sexes) maybe invoked to describe their sexual identity, as opposed to thinking of themselves as "gay" (which may be perceived to be a foreign term) [2]. A study conducted in Asia by Dowsett, Grierson, and McNally showed that the MSM population does not have similar traits other than being males and engaging in sex with other men [3]. The study concluded that the term MSM does not correspond to a single social identity. It refers to different behaviors and social identities [3, 4]. Public health researchers have sought to distinguish sexual orientation from sexual behaviors. In 2015, WHO estimated that the median HIV prevalence in MSM ranged from 4.3% in South East Asia to 14.9 percent in the African region [5].

Criminalization of consensual, adult same-sex behavior and stigma, discrimination, and violence against men who have sex with men has created an environment which compromises people's human rights [6]. To improve sustained, comprehensive, and effective HIV prevention, and testing and treatment efforts in low-, middle-, and high-income countries, WHO works closely with UNDP and UNAIDS to advocate for the implementation of a human rights-based approach for the prevention and treatment of HIV and sexually transmitted infections (STIs) [5]. The United States Department of Health and Human Services through the Affordable Care Act, 2012, offers new protection which includes preventing discrimination against lesbian, gay, bisexual, and transgender (LGBT) persons [7].

Funding is also provided for community-based preventive health programs and measures to combat HIV and related health problems.

Male homosexuality is associated with anal sex. However, MSM may also engage in oral sex or mutual masturbation. MSM face partner violence including by those with whom they engage in long-term, committed, emotional, and sexual relationships. Due to fear of stigmatization by medical professionals, MSM avoid seeking routine or appropriate health care. Physicians and other healthcare providers can help MSM overcome this barrier and improve health care of this community by being non-judgmental toward them.

2.2 Research on MSM

Research was undertaken to study the values, preferences, and practices with regard to self-care for sexual and reproductive health and rights (SRHR) and HIV prevention and treatment in men who have sex with men. The objectives were to understand their views about self-care practices; how they obtained information on self-care interventions; what were their motivations to use them; what barriers they faced while using them; and what they did if self-care practices failed.

Research was undertaken in Delhi, Mumbai, and Hyderabad. A qualitative research design was employed. In-depth interviews (IDIs), focus group discussions (FGDs), key informant interviews (KIIs), and workshops were conducted with men who have sex with men. Qualitative research methods allowed greater spontaneity and interaction with participants. They provided an opportunity to the participants to respond elaborately and in greater detail. The interviews were conducted using interview guides. The interviews were approximately 90–120 minutes in length. The interviews were recorded. The recordings were transcribed and checked for accuracy. Two IDIs, two KIs, and one FDG (8–10 participants) were conducted in Delhi and Mumbai each. One workshop (10 participants) was conducted in Delhi and one in Hyderabad (10 participants). The objective was to discuss self-care in MSM especially in relation to SRHR and HIV prevention. During the workshops, participants were provided with the canvas and paints and were asked to depict their sexual health practices in the form of paintings and artwork.

For the key informant interviews, participants were selected on the basis of their experience. They were peer educators working with NGOs. For in-depth interviews, outreach workers with 4–5 years of experience were selected. Focus group discussions included peer educators, outreach workers, and other young people. The data generated by KIs, IDIs, FGDs, and workshops were triangulated to obtain reliable information on these very complex issues.

Ethical approval for undertaking the study was granted by the Ethical Review Board of the Humsafar Trust. Before initiating the study, participants were given consent forms which described the study. Consent of all participants was taken on the forms and verbally. Confidentiality of participants was assured.

2.3 Research Findings

The findings include a discussion of the feelings and behaviors of MSM from childhood to adulthood; self-care interventions for SRHR; information sources for SRHR; risks and barriers faced by the community; and motivations for self-care.

2.3.1 An Expression of the Feelings and Behaviors of MSM

When they entered high school, around the age of 14–15 these young boys began to realize that they were more attracted to boys than to girls. Several signs appeared during their early childhood. When they were 4–5 years old, they liked to play with dolls and wanted to be with their mothers in the kitchen. They enjoyed dressing up in female attire and were interested in dancing and music. These interests enhanced their femininity. At this stage, they did not understand why they had different interests from other boys around them. They were unclear about their sexuality which made them very uncomfortable. Most of them did not understand the concept of homosexuality. They often fantasized about their own gender in their dreams.

> We fight with our own feelings to confirm our homogeneity.

Their mannerisms, socially perceived to be feminine, often manifested in effeminate body language which began to get noticed. They realized that stigma was associated with homosexuality. They felt distressed if anyone asked them about their sexual orientation. They hid their identity from their parents, families, and relatives. In their childhood, most experienced discrimination and bullying, which made them feel afraid.

> We feel afraid to show our feelings, people make fun of us and bully us.

People called them "*gur*" (homosexual). They were sexually abused by the older members of the family and the extended family and were then bribed and threatened to prevent them from telling anyone.

> They gave us chocolates and toys and sometimes threaten to put us in a dark room if we speak to anyone.

They wanted to talk about their sexual identity but were afraid to do so because of societal and parental disapproval.

> Our families are vehemently against us and ask us to hide our identity.

2.3.2 Self-care Interventions for Sexual and Reproductive Health

In the late 1990s and early 2000s, when there were few non-governmental organizations (NGOs) and the few that were there were not always accessible, information and awareness about sex and sexually were meager. Consequently, unprotected sex was a common feature. Now, almost all MSM are aware that they should use protective measures to prevent sexually transmitted infections (STIs). NGOs and peers have informed them about various interventions and have also made them realize the effectiveness of self-care.

> We got information about sexual health after we joined the NGO. They teach us how to maintain a healthy lifestyle.

The interventions they generally used were condoms and gels (Fig. 2.1). NGOs provided them information related to sexual and reproductive health. They received personal services from NGOs including regular medical checkups. They were tested for HIV, syphilis, and other STIs every three months. NGOs also provided them medicines and, if needed, referred them to the health centers for testing and treatment. MSM used self-testing kits distributed by NGOs. They used self-testing kits to check blood sugar and to test for STIs. They were not allowed to do HIV self-testing. They got this test done either at NGO centers or at the integrated counseling and testing centers (ICTCs).

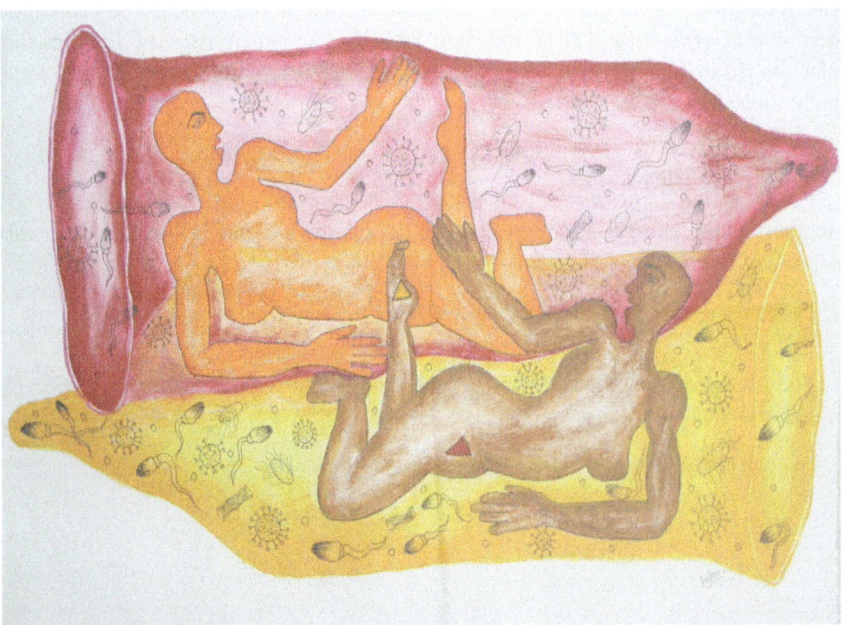

Fig. 2.1 Condoms for protection painting by Ashu (Bips)

2.3 Research Findings

> We are not allowed to test for HIV; NGOs do it for us.
>
> When the test is positive, NGOs send us to hospitals for reconfirmation.

NGOs and ICTCs provided pretest and posttest counseling for HIV.

To treat common ailments (flu, aches, pains, diarrhea), MSM got medicines from pharmacies. Those who could afford it got treatment for STIs from private practitioners. MSM did not visit government hospitals because of the high levels of stigma and discrimination they faced at these institutions. A qualified doctor, especially in a government setup, was most often the last resort.

> We face stigma and discrimination in government hospitals.
>
> Doctors do not treat us well, they are afraid to touch us. They take pictures of our genital parts for training young doctors and do not diagnose us properly.

MSM believed that they were at high risk of STIs. They developed oral ulcers and anal fissures. They most often sought advice about these conditions from their friends and peers. Those MSM who were associated with NGOs made contact with peer educators and outreach workers from the NGOs. Others went directly to pharmacies.

NGOs provided condoms and gels and also organized demonstrations to show them the correct use of condoms. NGOs conducted workshops to promote sexual and reproductive health. They addressed the sexual and reproductive health needs of MSM. They provided services and products such as contraceptives. They also provided information and knowledge on how to prevent illness and disease through role plays, dance, music, and other such activities. Some men preferred to obtain products such as condoms from NGOs.

Others were not averse to buying them from pharmacies. A key point to note is that men, by and large (to the extent of 80% during anal sex and 20% during oral sex), used condoms with "random" partners. However, this was not the case when they had sex with their regular or long-term partners (boyfriends).

2.3.3 Information Sources for Sexual and Reproductive Health

MSM believed that knowledge about sexual and reproductive health and HIV prevention was very important for them (Fig. 2.2). They obtained this information through social media, television, radio, and peer educators and NGO outreach workers. They got information through advertisements on sexual health, safe sex, and sexuality. They increasingly used the Internet for health information, dating, cybersex, and pornography. This technology also connected them to social networks of other MSM and bisexuals.

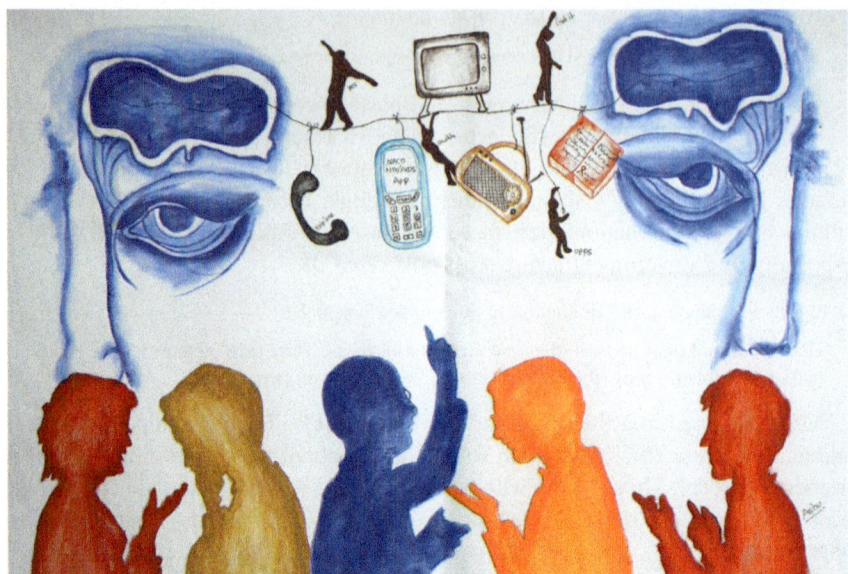

Fig. 2.2 Communicating the issues painting by Ashu (Bips)

NGO workers implemented behavior change communication activities to generate awareness about interventions for sexual and reproductive health. NGOs provided training to enable MSM to educate their peers on HIV prevention. They provided commodities such as condoms and lubricants and campaigned for better access to services by linking them to MSM-friendly HIV services. MSM also obtained information through pornographic magazines/films. They used different apps to get information related to sexual and reproductive health. These apps are specially designed for MSM to provide them with the information they need.

NGOs provided education on how to use pre-exposure prophylaxis (PrEP) to prevent HIV. So, they learned about PrEP. NGOs talked openly about condoms and safe sex. Therefore, MSM knew how to use condoms and were aware of their importance. They knew that they should wipe off the sperm or wash it with soap and water. If they ejaculated, they knew how to avoid getting the other's sperm or precum inside the anus and mouth. However, they did not know how to do HIV testing. Self-testing HIV kits are not available in the market. They are available in government hospitals and ICTCs and with NGOs conducting targeted interventions. These centers provide pre-test and post-test counseling. MSM were also linked with the community and used mobile apps that allowed them to network anonymously with community members in order to share information on STIs and HIV (infection and its prevention) and antiretroviral therapy (ART). They used helplines to obtain information about the treatment of infections. They used helplines to seek help regarding mental health problems which are highly prevalent among MSM.

2.3.4 Risks and Barriers Faced by the Community

Men who have sex with men are at increased risk of contracting HIV as well as other sexually transmitted infections. Some men in this study used shampoos, body lotions, and saliva instead of gels during penetrative sex, which caused redness, furuncles (boils), and irritation. Some were not able to read, so they at times used expired products. Some did not know the correct use of condoms. Others used double condoms in the belief that they will be better protected.

> We sometimes use two condoms during sex to make sure that no sperms penetrate and sometimes a condom is left inside.

Several MSM engaged in "chemsex" (commonly called party and play). They engaged with multiple sexual partners under the influence of psychoactive and performance enhancing drugs.

> We are generally in a monogamous relationship, but end up having sex with multiple partners when we are under the influence of drugs.

They used poppers (chemical drug substances) which led to multi-partner sex and increased the risk of STIs.

> We also use poppers which enhances our sexual contact with other men.

Many of the men engaged in casual sex and did not use condoms consistently. If they had small cuts or wounds, they were more vulnerable to HIV and STIs. Drugs and alcohol increased the risk of HIV. When they were under the influence of drugs and alcohol, they took more risks. Those who injected drugs often shared the same needles which increased the risk of STIs.

> We are not in our senses due to drugs, and so use the same needles.

Some did not know about water-based lubricants. They used petroleum jelly, body lotions or oils. Oil-based lubricants weaken latex condoms and cause them to break.

Many MSM were involved in paid sex from a very young age. They had unprotected sex to get extra money. Men who sold sex had more sexual partners and had more condomless sexual encounters.

> We agree to have sex without condom if they pay us double.

Some men who had sex with both men and women did not use condoms consistently with their female partners which resulted in transmission of infection to the latter.

> We generally do not use condoms with our wives. If we do, they think that either we have done something wrong or we have HIV.

These men got married under pressure from the family. They wanted to keep their sexual orientation secret due to stigma and so continued to have sex with their wives.

> My parents forced me to marry to keep their reputation in society even after they knew about my sexual orientation.

MSM had high rates of HIV. Many took antiretroviral therapy (ART), but adherence was a frequent problem.

2.3.5 Mental Health Issues Faced by the Community

MSM faced mental health issues of all kinds. Even though they are now becoming more accepted in society, there is still a stigma. People abused them, calling them names such as "*gur*" or "*hijra.*"

> Wherever we go, people insult us by calling us gur.

They faced a dilemma in revealing their sexual orientation to their families. They felt distressed because their sexuality was not condoned. They were not accepted by their families and had to hide their identity which caused stress, anxiety, and depression (Fig. 2.3). If they disclosed their identity, they faced stigma which led to low self-esteem. They were deprived of emotional support from their families. They faced stigma if they shared their sexual health problems with their families. Because their families did not support them, they often had to leave their homes. They then faced serious financial problems as they did not have stable jobs. They were constantly concerned about partner faithfulness which was a major cause of

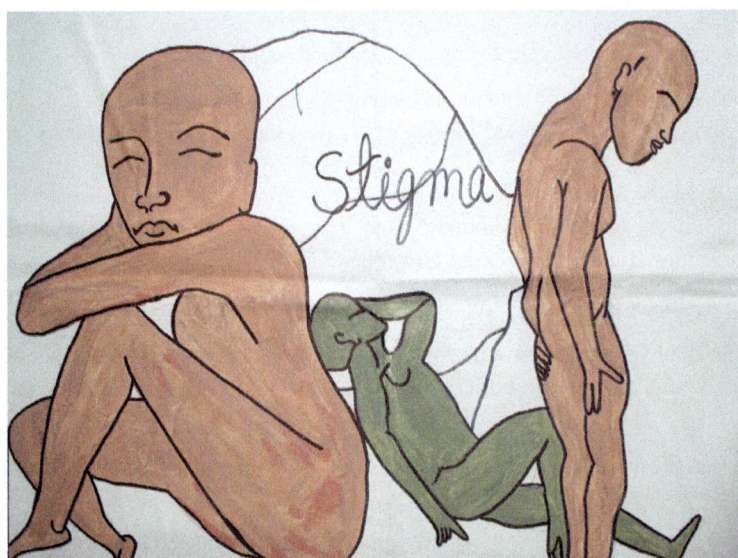

Fig. 2.3 Stigma faced by MSM painting by Ashu (Bips)

depression. They felt stressed because of rejection by the society and families which affected their mental health. Some committed suicide because they could not cope up with the stigma and discrimination that they faced.

2.3.6 Violence Faced by the Community

MSM faced (sexual, physical, and emotional) violence from family members, intimate partners, and clients, as well as from the police. If they were caught, the police harassed them and asked for money to let them go. They were also sexually harassed by the police.

> Police harass us and asks us for money if they catch us in the washroom or even with condoms. If we refuse they beat us, put us in prison. Some policemen also take advantage of us.

They were bullied by members of their families, peers in school, and by society in general. They faced sexual harassment by their families at a very young age. They also faced intimate partner violence. Their partners tortured and abused them physically, mentally, and financially.

> Our partners torture us and ask us for money. They take us for granted. They beat us if we refuse to give them money.

In healthcare settings also MSM experienced discrimination, judgmental attitude, and breach of confidentiality. The doctors took pictures of their genitalia and used these for medical education. They were often stripped and used as specimens to demonstrate STIs in teaching institutions.

> Doctors are afraid of touching us. They take pictures of our genitalia for teaching.

2.3.7 Motivation for Self-care

MSM were at high risk of STI and HIV infection. Earlier, they were unaware about the risks of unprotected sex and had limited knowledge, so they took risks and suffered the consequences. Over the years, with greater awareness provided by NGOs and with the development and advancement in technology and social media, they are now far more aware of their risks. There are effective health education programs by the NGOs to promote self-care practices among MSM. MSM get free condoms and other self-care products from NGOs. They can visit healthcare facilities for ART treatment. Since they are aware of the risks they face and can also access health services, they feel motivated to use interventions for prevention and treatment.

> The level of awareness and information inspired us to do self-care.

Better information and technology have enhanced awareness. Programs by NGOs and government to bring about positive behavior change have made a difference. MSM are now moving towards a positive lifestyle to improve their quality of life. Since they have more information, they are better able to practice self-care which has become an important aspect of their lives.

2.4 From Vulnerability to Resilience

2.4.1 MSM's Personal Narrative on Self-care

Documented By: Dr. Rashmi Pachauri Rajan

For men who have sex with men, within the context of sexual and reproductive health and HIV prevention, what does self-care mean?

This is the story of Bips, a 41-year-old man, born to a South Indian middle-class family, originally from a village called Marambalyam near Salem in the state of Tamil Nadu in India. He was, however, born and brought up in Delhi. His father was in a transferable job, so traveled extensively, while his mother stayed in Delhi and looked after the family while she also worked as a maid. Bips grew up with five older sisters.

He was his parent's only living son as several children had died in infancy. He was born after much prayer and anxiety, given the culture of patriarchy and son preference in India. Therefore, he was considered precious and was always over-protected. He was the only one among his siblings who completed school and was educated.

As he was growing up, he was also growing more and more feminine. He was molly-coddled by his mother and sisters and grew up playing "dress-up" and "dolls" with them. He enjoyed dressing up in girls' clothes. Before his *mundan* ceremony—a religious ceremony where all the hair is shaved off as an offering to God to purify the child and keep away the evil eye—he had long hair which, along with his sisters, his mother would oil and plait every night before bed.

In 1984, when Indira Gandhi was assassinated and riots broke out in Delhi, Bips was six years old. Since their household consisted of him, his five sisters, and his mother (his father being away on work much of the year), his mother felt the need of a male family member as a means of protection for the family. She requested her sister to allow her son (a young man) to stay with them, a request that was granted. This arrangement continued for a while. It was some time after this that a friend of his cousin began coming to their house. It started with him placing Bips on his knee and playing with and cuddling and kissing him. This gradually took a more amorous turn and finally took the shape of sexual assault on Bips. Even as the small child he was then, Bips knew there was something very wrong and "bad" which he did not like, but was totally helpless to stop. He knew that if he complained, the young man would deny it and his word would be believed. And so, Bips kept quiet.

However, surprisingly, when this young man left, Bips "missed" the "feelings" that his touch and caresses used to evoke in him!

Bips began to realize that he was more attracted to men and this enhanced his feminine characteristics even more—resulting in changes in his demeanor, dressing, and body language. And because of this, he began to experience discrimination, bullying, and isolation. He knew nothing about homosexuality, and there was no one with whom he could discuss these feelings and emotions. And soon, not just outsiders but even the extended family began commenting on his behavior and demeanor, calling him a *hijra* (eunuch), which was extremely hurtful. This was also reason enough for Bips father to get physically abusive and violent with him. And this led to bouts of depression and feelings of isolation for Bips.

However, Bips also realized that, much as he was pressured by his parents to take his studies seriously (to the exclusion of all else), what he really enjoyed and was getting very good at was art, music, and dancing. He began concentrating on these activities, much to the disapproval and anger of his parents and family. In fact, at one stage, he secretly got a job washing cars so he could take a course in art and painting, which he enjoyed thoroughly, learned a lot from, and got quite adept at.

It was around this stage in his life when he started noticing people "like himself" more and more. And through increased contact with his new-found friends, he was introduced to a group of men who have sex with men (MSM) who met once a week at the *Hanuman Mandir* near Connaught Place. And that was his coming of age!

"Oh my God, this is our place… why didn't I come here before" was the thought in his mind as his eyes grew wide with wonder and delight. *"They are my family, I am able to understand them, feel their laugh and relate to their experiences."*

Even though he was still strictly monitored with respect to his freedom to leave the house, he managed to find time to meet his friends and interact with the MSM community. And all the while, his sexual orientation became more and more clear to him, in which he began to revel.

Through the MSM community, he met outreach workers of the Naz Foundation, a non-governmental organization (NGO) that works on HIV/AIDS and sexual health. At Naz, he was introduced for the first time to condoms. He also began to gain more and more information about sexual and reproductive health, including HIV prevention, particularly pertaining to gay men and transgender. Bips decided at that stage that he wanted to get involved in social work.

Through his years growing up, Bips' family went through a lot of hardship and family conflict, which affected the time and emotion his parents were able to devote to their children. His father was estranged from his brothers. Bips lost a sister through domestic violence, while another was divorced. He found solace for a while in Christianity and in his art. But because of the nature of the sorrow and trauma these incidents had caused during this period, he underwent severe depression. With advice from friends and family, he tried meditation, reading, socializing, taking calcium and vitamins, and exercising. At that time, Internet had not come into its own and there was not enough relevant and authentic information available or accessible on mental health. Finally, he consulted a doctor who prescribed a three-month course of medication. He also put himself on sleeping pills for a short period of time as he was sleep deprived. And in time, he felt mentally well and strong again, and stopped the medication.

Bips was later "married" to a man. But this relationship was violent and distressing while it lasted, and ended after a couple of years. Depression once again reared its ugly head. However, this time Bips self-medicated based on his earlier experience. And over time, he learned to discipline his mind and body. He now prides himself for being a "mentally strong" person, who has learned from his bad experiences.

> I have faced many forms of violence – sexual harassment, domestic violence, partner violence, and violence from the police – but I am now a mentally strong person.

It was then that he applied as a social worker at the Naz Foundation and got a job there as an outreach worker. He worked diligently and, in the process, learned and enhanced his levels of information. He trained as a counselor, as a master trainer, and as an outreach worker. However, wonderful as this experience was, along with his colleagues he was regularly harassed violently and sexually by the police and the local dons. It seemed to be a part and parcel of the life of a gay man. But Bips felt passionate about his work and his zeal to help others remained high, no matter what hardships he endured. And in spite of the violence and the harassment he regularly faced, Bips was enjoying his work, his life, and his sexuality.

And it was then that pressure started building up by his family to get married. Fearful of disclosing his sexuality to his family, Bips got married to a young woman his family selected for him. The marriage was not consummated and resulted in somewhat of a messy divorce a few months later.

Bips continued his work with the Naz Foundation. But on one occasion when he was being beaten and harassed by police, some police officers who were from his locality happened to see him. They went to his home and informed his parents that their son was gay. After a lot of angry and heartbreaking words, violence, resentment, and tears, although it took time, his parents eventually accepted his sexual orientation and accepted their son for what he is.

Bips has had a long and difficult life journey as a young, gay man. Through his own life experiences as well as what he learned formally in his profession, he is well informed and knowledgeable about self-care for the promotion of his sexual and reproductive health, and the prevention of HIV.

> I am a trainer, counselor, and coordinator....

Over time, he has disciplined himself about his diet, lifestyle (exercise, meditation, medications, allopathic as well as herbal, etc.), protection, and safe sex. He is tech-savvy and procures information as and when required, from the Internet and from various Apps, as well as from several NGOs.

> I have 300 Apps on my phone.

He is educated and so is able to read, comprehend, and use pamphlets. He can understand instructions on medications he buys. With regard to sources of information, Bips feels that television and radio, though they do provide information related to sexually transmitted infections and HIV as well as family planning, are not really useful as they do not provide sufficient or detailed information, because of censorship. He feels that the information that TV and the radio give is more male-centric and does not provide adequate and appropriate information for women.

Bips has faith in doctors. He shared his perspective saying that it is very important that when there is a health issue, the appropriate specialist should be consulted, and not just any general physician, because the specialist will be able to diagnose the problem and prescribe the relevant medication. His concern, however, is that very often doctors, though educated, are insensitive, judgmental, and discriminatory, especially when dealing with MSM, transgender, and the socially and economically lower classes. And ironically and unfortunately, it is these disadvantaged and marginalized sections of society that do not have the means (education or accessibility) for obtaining appropriate self-care. And then of course, there are always times when a doctor is not available or accessible and self-care is the only course to take.

Bips has worked with NGOs and interacted intensively personally and professionally with health professionals. So, he is knowledgeable about the more common sexually transmitted infections (STIs) and related problems. He, therefore, knows which symptoms require what medication. He often self-medicates and, in fact, also provides information and advice to his family, friends, and colleagues with regard to their health. He also advises them about when they should consult a doctor or a specialist, if he feels the problem is serious and professional intervention is needed.

Bips keeps detailed notes of medications (oral as well as creams and gels) and the dosages he has used in the past which have been prescribed by a doctor. Whenever he suffers from similar problems, he follows the same regimen again. He often advises friends who have similar health issues and tells them about the medication they need.

With respect to HIV prevention and, specifically, regarding self-testing kits for HIV diagnosis, Bips has very strong views. He feels that although HIV self-testing kits instructions for use that is not nearly enough. HIV testing definitely requires pre- and posttest counseling which is lacking when doing a self-test. Nor is it mentioned anywhere in the HIV self-test kit that counseling is a must before and after the test. This, Bips feels, is dangerous and insensitive, as a positive result could lead to serious mental health problems such as depression and even suicide.

> There should be a helpline number on the pamphlet where the steps are written for use. If an NGO is providing it, they will do counseling, but if it is from a chemist shop, there should be helpline number of an NGO so that they can take counseling, if not before testing, then at least after testing.

Speaking for himself, and having worked with NGOs and interacted closely with doctors, he is well aware of the myths and misconceptions surrounding the spread of STIs in general and HIV in particular. However, he refrains from anal sex and has, in fact, done so for years (he had a bad experience once when a condom burst). And he feels that he will only "allow" anal penetration if he finds a partner with whom he shares emotional, mental as well as physical compatibility. Meantime, indulging in foreplay, body play, and oral sex is sufficient. But now having much more knowledge about the importance of condoms, he always uses condoms (of good quality, no matter what the price), as he feels that it is one of the most important methods of safe sex and self-care for his lifestyle—for gay men, he says, HIV infection has a high risk of spreading via anal sex.

Bips spoke about issues of accountability when self-care fails. Within the formal healthcare system of doctors and clinics, it is easy to go back to the doctor and get medicines or dosages changed if a problem occurs or persists or if there are adverse side effects. However, if information has been obtained from the Internet and the intervention has not worked for some reason, he feels he is knowledgeable and smart enough to be able to go to other sites or apps to get more information and alternative solutions to deal with his problem. It is only when that also does not work that he consults a doctor. This is the advice he follows both for himself and for his family (his mother, sisters, nieces, and nephews) and friends, who often come to him with their health and other problems.

Life has finally taken a new and peaceful turn for Bips, after years of trauma and conflict, both internally and from the family and the wider community. After constant financial and personal hardship, family conflicts, and keeping secrets, Bips is now at peace with his family. His family and friends have accepted his sexuality and respect him for his strengths and talents. He is asked for assistance and information, ranging from topics related to marriage, makeup, hair styles, to helping with advice on medicines, health in general, and sexual and reproductive health in particular. He has aspirations in the long term to adopt a child and, in fact, to eventually undergo a sex change.

So again, what does self-care mean for Bips?

> …it is a process where we can keep ourselves fit and safe from diseases, and if something happens, then we have the means and the knowledge to give ourselves relief. We should be aware that even though there are benefits we get from self-care and self-intervention, there can be harm too. We should proceed with self-care keeping in view both its advantages and disadvantages.

2.5 Discussion

Self-care holds great promise for men who have sex with men, a hard-to-reach minority community that is at high risk of HIV infection and is especially vulnerable. The term MSM was defined by the US Centers for Disease Control and Prevention in 2007 as "all men who have sex with other men, regardless of how they identify themselves (gay, bisexual, or heterosexual)." In India, the term MSM encompasses many identities, gender constructs, and communities. It includes a wide range of distinct categories of men who self-identify themselves as gay, bisexual, transgender, or heterosexual and engage in sex with other men [8]. MSM is a term that is used to present a very complex dynamic in a simplified way [9]. This term, however, fails to convey identities and behaviors of these men.

2.5 Discussion

MSM in India can be categorized into various subgroups [10]. One group includes mostly self-identified and behaviorally homosexual men. Allegedly effeminate men who are thought to be the penetrated partners self-identify themselves as *kothis* or *dangas*. In spite of this label, they often penetrate other men (*dhoru-kothis*) and may also be married and engage in vaginal intercourse. The male partners of *kothis* are named *panthis* or *giriyas*—"the real man." This label is often provided by the person who is being penetrated by him [11]. A study of *kothi* identified MSM in West Bengal revealed that there is a distinction in the educational and economic status of the different MSM categories where gender attitude difference prevailed prominently. *Ariyal kothis* and *hijras* have lower formal education than other groups but in case of income *ariyal kothis* ranked lower than other groups [8].

Asthana and Oostvogels reported that *kothis* may find it difficult to negotiate safe sex with *panthis* due to the fear of losing them. Some MSM identify themselves as gay, conforming to the Western identity structure. Often, these men will have a coming out process comparable to the one experienced in the West [12].

Boyce emphasized that "National foundation for India (NFI) policy and practice is deliberately positioned in contradistinction to what the organization posits as an ostensibly Westernized mode of gay identification, characteristic of an urban, internationalist Indian social milieu, filtered through the diaspora, but which is seen as largely irrelevant to the majority of men who have sex with men (NFI 2000, 2003)" [9].

Earlier programs for MSM did not incorporate the issues of rights or questions of identity. These complexities were sidelined. As programming to prevent and treat sexually transmitted infections including HIV matures, it should incorporate these important facets. Previously receiving little attention, MSM are now increasingly being recognized in India as a group that is at increased risk for HIV and other STIs [13]. The link between sexual identity and sexual behavior is a complex phenomenon strongly embedded in a very specific context in India [14–16]. By some, male–male sex among "heterosexually" identified men is often not considered as "sex" per se. It is referred to as *masti* or fun between men [17, 18].

It is imperative that doctors ask all MSM clients in an open and non-judgmental way about their sexual behavior and provide routine HIV testing and STI screening and treatment. Doctors should be comfortable to routinely ask about sexual practices, focusing on what the client does, rather than how he identify himself.

A risk group that recently gained importance in HIV prevention programs in India consists of male sex workers. These men are at high risk of acquiring HIV infection [19–21]. The population groups commonly involved in male sex work in India, particularly in urban centers such as Mumbai, are masseurs at train stations, beaches, or in some massage parlors; transgender in prostitution practicing male sex work in their homes or near truck terminuses or specific sites on highways; physical instructors in gymnasium; young migrant males practicing male sex for survival; and college students and men with other occupations practicing male sex work for extra money [20, 22].

Finally, another important subgroup is married MSM [23, 24]. Although this group may cut across many other subgroups including self-identified MSM, non-identified MSM, HIV-infected MSM, non-infected MSM, men in sex work, and even male-to-female transgender, these men require specific interventions. They may be more likely to be older compared to unmarried MSM and have anonymous hurried sex with a stranger due to the fear of being found out in social settings. These married MSM may potentially have difficulty in discussing their infection and their sexuality with their spouses. They also have feelings of guilt due to sexual encounters out of marriage. It is important to understand these issues in order to intervene effectively for the prevention of HIV and STIs in these men.

Given the need of confidentiality that is of critical importance for MSM, self-care has special meaning in their lives. Healthcare providers need to understand the different categories of MSM to intervene effectively. NGOs are playing an important role in addressing the problems of STIs including HIV as they have a greater understanding of the sexual behaviors of different subgroups of MSM. NGOs are also closer to these communities and have their trust. NGOs can, therefore, be significant players in promoting and supporting self-care practices among MSM. Increasing access to technology is also facilitating self-care among them.

Literature on self-care by MSM is currently almost nonexistent. Our research shows encouraging results. However, much more research is needed to assess how self-care in MSM can be enhanced. The potential to increase self-care in men who have sex with men is considerable with the increased availability of self-care technologies and the rapidly increasing social media which can not only provide more information on self-care but can also increase the pace of interaction between MSM networks, thereby accelerating the diffusion of information across geographies.

References

1. UNAIDS: Men who have sex with men. United Nations. 2006.
2. Patel VV, Mayer KH, Makadon HJ. Men who have sex with men in India: A diverse population in need of medical attention. Indian J Med Res. 2012;136(4):563–70.
3. Dowsett G, Grierson J, McNally S. A review of knowledge about the sexual networks and behaviors of men who have sex with men in Asia. Aust Res Centre Sex Health Soc Melbourne Australia;2006 May.
4. Guttmacher Institute. Patterns of men's use of sexual and reproductive health services. 2007.
5. World Health Organization. Men who have sex with men. WHO/HIV/2015.8. World Health Organization, Geneva;2015 October.
6. World Health Organization. Health education service. Health education in self-care: Possibilities and limitations. World Health Organization, Geneva; 1984. Report No.: HED/84.1.
7. The Affordable Care Act Helps LGBT Americans. 2017 March.
8. Dey S, Das A. Difference in education and income status of the kothi identified MSM of West Bengal, India. Int J Res. 2015;2(2):574–88.
9. Mcnally SP, Dowsett GW, Grierson JW. MSM-A catch-all term that may not catch enough: Rethinking MSM epidemiology and prevention in Asia following a review of MSM research in four countries. Paper presented at XV International Conference on AIDS, Bangkok, Thailand;2004.

References

10. Robertson J. Case study: The Humsafar Trust, Mumbai, India: Empowering communities of men who have sex with men to prevent HIV. Arlington, VA: USAID AIDS Support and Technical Assistance Resources, AIDSTAR-One Task order 1. 2010.
11. Chan R, Kavi AR, Carl G, Khan S, Oetomo D, Tan ML, Brown T. HIV and men who have sex with men: Perspectives from selected Asian countries. AIDS. 1998;12(B):59–65, 67–8.
12. Bhugra D, Rahman Q, Bhintade R. Sexual fantasy in gay men in India: A comparison with heterosexual men. Sex Relatsh Ther. 2006;21:197–207.
13. Verma R, Shekhar A, Khobragade S, Adhikary R, George B, Ramesh BM, Ranebennur V, Mondal S, Patra RK, Srinivasan S, Vijayaraman A, Paul SR, Bohidar N. Scale-up and coverage of Avahan: A large-scale HIV-prevention programme among female sex workers and men who have sex with men in four Indian states. Sex Transm Infect. 2010;86(1):76–82.
14. Asthana S, Oostvogels R. The social construction of male "homosexuality" in India: Implications for HIV transmission and prevention. Soc Sci Med. 2001;52:707–21.
15. Khan S. Culture, sexualities, and identities. J Homosex. 2001;40(3–4):99–115.
16. Pappas G, Khan O, Wright TJ, Khan S, Kumaramnagalam L, O'Neill J. Males who have sex with males and HIV/AIDS in India: The hidden epidemic. AIDS Public Policy J. 2001;16:4–17.
17. Dandona L, Dandona R, Gutierrez JP, Kumar GA, McPherson S, Bertozzi SM. Sex behavior of men who have sex with men and risk of HIV in Andhra Pradesh, India. AIDS. 2005;19:611–9.
18. Sengupta S, Verma K, Bhattacharya S, Banerjee A. Economic, political, social and cultural determinants of high-risk behavior amongst groups at heightened risk of STD/HIV infection. Paper presented at the XII International Conference on AIDS, Geneva, Switzerland;1998 June–July.
19. Chakrapani V. Aravanis [Hijras/Alis] in sex work in Chennai. Paper presented at the First National Conference of the Network of Male Sex Workers, Thiruvananthapuram, India;2003a March.
20. Chakrapani V. Male sex work in Chennai [India]. Paper presented at the First National Conference of the Network of Male Sex Workers, Thiruvananthapuram, India;2003b March.
21. Dandona L, Dandona R, Kumar GA, Gutierrez JP, McPherson S, Bertozzi SM & the ASCI FPP Study Team. How much attention is needed towards men who sell sex to men for HIV prevention in India? BMC Public Health. 2006 Feb;15;6(1):31.
22. Row Kavi A. Reaching out. India: Beyond the monsoon. AIDS Action. 1991;15, 4.
23. Gurha S. Social determinants of behavior: Indian society has some of the most unique social constraints. Paper presented at the 12th International Conference on AIDS, Geneva, Switzerland;1998 June–July.
24. Khan M, Menon S, Kumar ML. The significance of married MSM in HIV/AIDS prevention. Paper presented at the International Conference on AIDS, Durban, South Africa;2000 July.

Open Access This chapter is licensed under the terms of the Creative Commons Attribution 4.0 International License (http://creativecommons.org/licenses/by/4.0/), which permits use, sharing, adaptation, distribution and reproduction in any medium or format, as long as you give appropriate credit to the original author(s) and the source, provide a link to the Creative Commons license and indicate if changes were made.

The images or other third party material in this chapter are included in the chapter's Creative Commons license, unless indicated otherwise in a credit line to the material. If material is not included in the chapter's Creative Commons license and your intended use is not permitted by statutory regulation or exceeds the permitted use, you will need to obtain permission directly from the copyright holder.

Chapter 3
Understanding Health Needs of Transgender

3.1 Backdrop

Transgenders are individuals whose gender identity does not conform to gender norms and expectations traditionally associated with their sex assigned at birth [1]. It is an identity or expression when gender differs from sex. Those who have medical interventions to transition from one sex to another identify as transsexuals. The term transgender includes people who belong to the third gender. The terms transgender and transsexual are commonly based on distinctions between gender (psychological and social) and sex (physical) [2, 3]. Transsexuality may be said to deal more with physical aspects of one's sex, while transgender relates more to one's psychological gender disposition or predisposition [4].

> According to WHO, transgender have lower access to health and HIV services due to a range of issues including legal barriers and stigma and discrimination. WHO works with international and country partners to address the varied health needs of transgender, including HIV prevention, diagnosis and treatment and also to address structural barriers which impact service access by transgender [5].

A lack of legal recognition of transgender in most countries contributes to their exclusion and marginalization. Transwomen are around 49 times more likely to be living with HIV than other adults of reproductive age with an estimated worldwide HIV prevalence of 19 percent. A 2008 synthesis of published US studies reported that HIV rates among Black, White, and Hispanic transwomen (assigned male at birth) was 56%, 17%, and 16%, respectively. HIV infection rates among transmen (assigned female at birth) have been difficult to determine [6].

In some countries, HIV prevalence in transwomen is 80 times more than the general adult population. The United States National HIV/AIDS Strategy notes that transgenders are at high risk for HIV infection and efforts specifically targeting transgender populations are minimal. Transgender adults and adolescents, regardless of HIV rates, have many individual, interpersonal, social, and structural factors contributing to HIV infection risk, not all of which are unique to their gender identity [6].

A comprehensive package of services is recommended to address HIV in transgender through health interventions for injected drugs, HIV testing and counseling, HIV treatment and care, and sexual and reproductive health [5].

In the early twentieth century, cross-dressing and transgender and gender non-conforming (TGNC) were medicalized. John Hopkins University started providing gender-affirming care followed by University of Minnesota and other medical centers across the USA [7]. In the 1980s and 1990s, clinical services were primarily provided in private practice. Some transgender health research was being conducted in the USA. A surge in research followed which revealed that TGNC people are disproportionately affected by HIV.

Many transgenders experience gender dysphoria and seek medical treatment such as hormone replacement, surgery, and psychotherapy [8]. All transgenders do not desire such treatment, but some who do cannot undergo sex reassignment surgery (SRS) because of financial or medical reasons [8, 9].

Many transgenders face discrimination in the workplace and in accessing public accommodations and health care. Also, in most places, they are not legally protected from discrimination [10–12]. Non-recognition of identity of transgender results in their facing extreme discrimination in all spheres of society, especially in the fields of employment, education, and health care.

Despite the discrimination between sexual orientation and gender, throughout history, the gay, lesbian, and bisexual subculture was often the only place where gender-variant people were socially accepted in the gender role they felt they belonged to, especially during the time when legal or medical transitioning was almost impossible.

3.2 Research on Transgender

Research was undertaken to study the values, preferences, and practices with regard to self-care for sexual and reproductive health and rights (SRHR) and HIV prevention and treatment in transgender. The objectives were to obtain an understanding of their views about self-care practices; how they obtained information on self-care interventions; what were their motivations to use them; what barriers they faced while using them; and what they did if self-care practices failed.

Research was undertaken in Delhi, Mumbai, Hyderabad, and Coimbatore. A qualitative study design was employed. In-depth interviews (IDIs), focus group discussions (FGDs), key informant interviews (KIIs), and workshops were conducted with transgender. Qualitative research methods allowed greater spontaneity and interaction with participants. They provided an opportunity to the participants to respond elaborately and in greater detail. The interviews were conducted using interview guides. The interviews were approximately 90–120 minutes in length. The interviews were recorded, and the recordings were transcribed and checked for accuracy. Two IDIs, two KIIs, and one FGD (8–10 participants) were conducted in Mumbai. Workshops were conducted with 10 participants each in Delhi, Hyderabad, and Coimbatore to understand their general health problems, sexual health, and HIV, and how they accessed information on SRH products and services on social media and other platforms.

For the key informant interviews, participants were selected on the basis of their experience. They were peer educators working with NGOs. For in-depth interviews, outreach workers with 4–5 years of experience were selected. Focus group discussions included peer educators, outreach workers, and other young people. During the workshop, participants were asked to depict their sexual practices in art form for which they were provided with colors and canvas.

Triangulation of data generated by KIIs, IDIs, FGDs, and workshops made it possible to obtain reliable information on complex issues. Ethical approval for undertaking the study was granted by the Ethical Review Board of the Humsafar Trust. Before initiating the study, participants were given consent forms which described the study. Consent of all participants was taken in writing and orally. Confidentiality of all participants was assured.

3.2.1 Research Findings

The findings include a discussion of the feelings and behaviors of transgender from childhood to adulthood; self-care interventions for SRHR; information sources for SRHR; risks and barriers faced by the community; and motivations for self-care.

3.2.2 Reflections of Transgender

> Having the soul of a woman and body of a man… it is like a woman is trapped in a man's body' and it kills a person from the inside.

They had this feeling from their childhood but when they turned around seven, they began to perceive effeminate feelings. Most transgender started realizing that they were different from their brothers and other men around.

> During our childhood, we liked to play with dolls and were more involved in household work with our mothers.

They were physically abused at an early age by family members and other men.

> After abusing us physically, the older members of the family forced us to keep silent.

Some of them were very keen to undergo their sexual transition partly or fully. In this process, they faced many difficulties.

> If we have soul of a woman, we want to look like a woman.

Some wanted to undergo sexual transition, but their families did not agree because of societal discrimination and status within their community.

> After knowing my identity, my family wanted to hide it from society and forced me to behave and dress like a man.

Most of them eventually left their families and began living alone or among other transgender. Their *"gurus"* (teachers) and other transgender were their only support system. They were their only family.

> Only the gurus support us and allow us to live as we are.

3.2.3 Self-care Interventions for Sexual and Reproductive Health

With respect to self-care interventions, they preferred to use condoms and gels. Either they got these free of cost from NGOs or their clients brought them along. The use of gels was very common among transgender. They sometimes purchased these from medical stores, although that was not always affordable.

> Due to lack of money, sometimes we cannot even buy a condom.

The study indicates that earlier when they were not aware of the risks of unprotected sex they were ready to have sexual encounters without protection (Fig. 3.1). This is now not the case and most used condoms and gels during penetrative sex. However, transgender did not always use condoms during sex with long-term partners ("boyfriends" or "husbands").

They frequently had sex without protection for the sake of more money.

> We easily get ready for sex without condoms for extra money.

They were reportedly violated by their clients and were forced to have unprotected sex.

> It is more important for us to live than to insist on the use of condoms when a client is threatening.

The study showed that they required more comprehensive interventions for sexual and reproductive health. To treat common ailments (flu, aches, pains, diarrhea), the community often visited known pharmacists for medication. Those who could afford to visit private practitioners for HIV and STI treatment did so. Many who could not afford treatment from qualified medical practitioners visited quacks and untrained practitioners. This community visited the government hospital, as a last resort. This was because of the high levels of stigma and discrimination they faced at government hospitals, especially for treatment of sexually transmitted infections (STIs) and HIV. The hospitals and centers provided antiretroviral therapy (ART). There have been technological innovations and

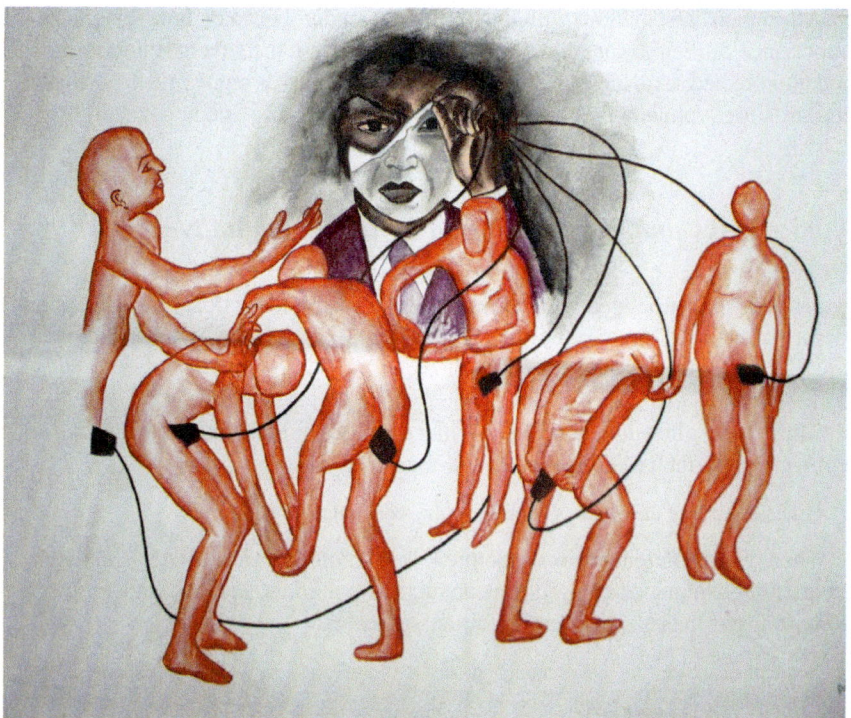

Fig. 3.1 Unsafe sex with multiple partners painting by Ashu (Bips)

developments in medical technologies. Transgenders, however, feel deprived as they could not get these products because of their inability to pay for them. The study showed that because of lack of social support, limited resources, and fear of violence, transgenders had to compromise their sexual health.

3.2.4 *Information Sources for Sexual and Reproductive Health*

The data revealed that transgender had knowledge about sexual and reproductive health. They got information about protected and safe sex through the social media, mass media, television, radio, and peer educators and NGO outreach workers. NGOs organized workshops and undertook behavior change communication activities to enhance the communities' knowledge and to make them better informed about sexual and reproductive health products and services.

>NGOs provide us information through workshops and outreach workers.

After their association with NGOs, transgender became more aware of the importance of their sexual and reproductive health and the adverse effects of unsafe and unprotected sex. NGOs provided them services such as regular medical checkups and tests for syphilis, other STIs and HIV. NGOs also provided counseling.

3.2.5 Risks and Barriers Faced by the Community

Some transgender begged in local trains and at road intersections. They were given targets of earnings per day by their *gurus.*

> We have to earn 1000 bucks a day.

They were often not allowed to enter the local trains and were beaten up or thrown out by the police if they found them begging.

> Police beats us if they find us begging in the local trains.

There were different socio-economic levels among the transgender. Some did not have enough money to buy products such as condoms, creams, and gels, which compromised their sexual and reproductive health.

> Sometimes we do not have enough money to buy food, condoms and gels are just a thought.

There were many transgender who provided economical and emotional support to their families and even to the families of their partners.

> We are responsible for taking care of the needs of our family. It is a part of our struggle which we have accepted.

After their association with the NGOs, they became more aware of the adverse effects of unprotected sex and refused to have sexual encounters without protection.

> We are well informed now. We do not have sex without using condoms.

A number of transgender opted to undergo transition partly or fully. Some used hormones without medical consultation and advice which led to complications and had adverse effects on their health. However, over time, they became more aware of the importance of professional services. They underwent the procedures for gender transition through medical channels.

The study showed that transgender faced multiple obstacles in accessing government health services. These included discrimination and refusal of treatment. They were stigmatized, so they preferred to take medicines from the pharmacies. Sometimes, they were not able to explain their sexual health problems to the pharmacist and so took inappropriate medications, which resulted in side-effects and other health problems.

> We do not clearly explain our sexual health problems and sometimes take the wrong medication.

Breast enhancement

Peers suggested various drugs that had worked for them for breast enhancement. They obtained these drugs from known pharmacists. The risk of taking unprescribed medication (often in the wrong doses) resulted in complications, including kidney and liver disease. Their extreme gender dysphoria compelled them to transition, for which they needed surgery and hormones, at any cost. A critical factor when making decisions about transitioning was the cost of interventions. Though more expensive, those who could afford them preferred using silicone breast implants because they were reportedly safer. However, the community described several instances of silicon packing shifting out-of-place and leading to severe pain and other complications.

The community also went to great lengths to develop large nipples by using methods suggested by their peers and their *gurus,* which often resulted in severe complications. The community felt it lacked reliable information regarding its transitioning needs. Given the high costs of transitioning, they were often forced into sex work to raise the money to pay for hormones and surgery. They also spent a great deal of money on beauty products and treatment (Fig. 3.2). Based on advice received from their peers and *gurus*, they bought creams, jellies, and injections from pharmacists (they knew and regularly visited) to support their transition. They also bought products such as condoms, lubes, sex toys, and sex enhancement drugs online using the Internet.

Sex Reassignment Surgery

The community primarily sought information on sex reassignment surgery (SRS) from peers and *gurus*. There were only a few qualified medical practitioners who carried out SRS. Even among those who were qualified, many were unable to deal with postoperative complications.

> I was left with a hanging tube and bag for urine, which required frequent intervention because the tube detached itself and professional help was needed to reinstate it.

Additionally, qualified doctors often charged prohibitive prices making them inaccessible to most members of the community. For those who could not afford expensive doctors, unqualified practitioners and quacks were the only option. Unqualified practitioners conducted procedures under unhygienic conditions, without sterilization which resulted in infections, other complications, and even death.

3.2.6 Violence Faced by the Community

Those infected with HIV often lacked information about their condition and how to treat it. Since many had little or no information about their condition, they frequently dropped out of ART treatment. They faced stigma and discrimination in

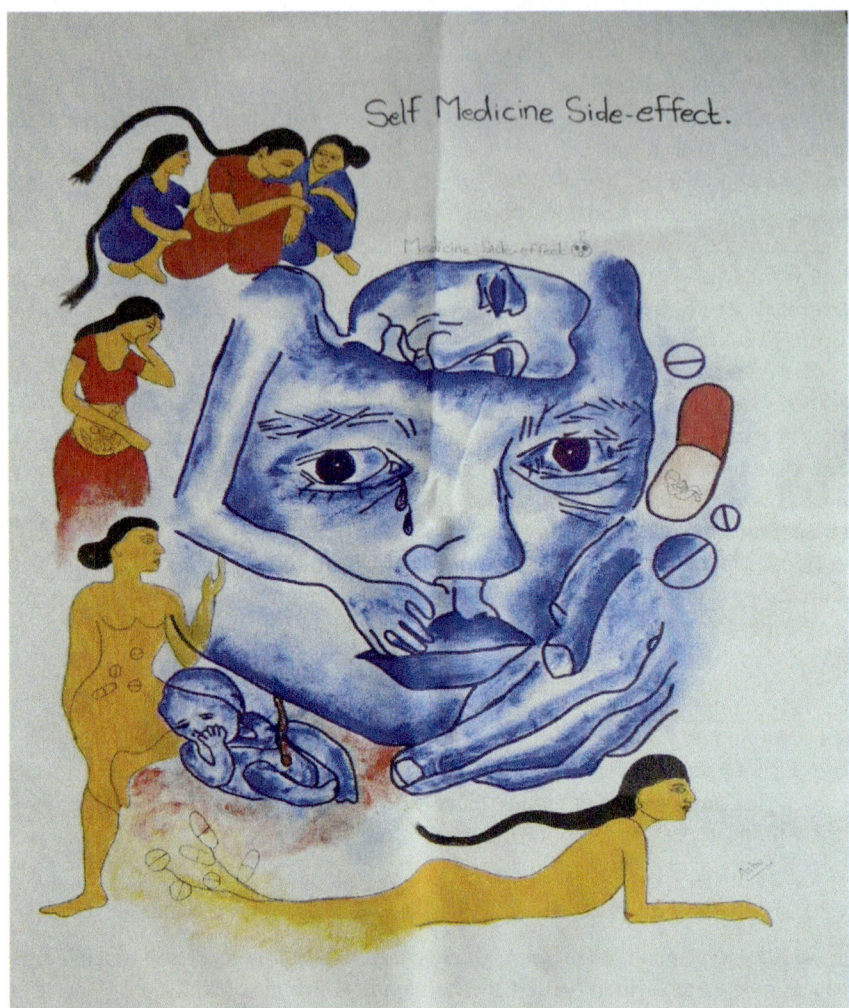

Fig. 3.2 Enhancing beauty painting by Ashu (Bips)

government hospitals. The junior doctors were not experienced with treating STIs in the community. They were often stripped and used as specimens to demonstrate different STIs in teaching institutions. They were verbally abused. They were treated as "untouchables" and examined from afar.

> Doctors take pictures of our genitalia and show them to the senior doctors for medical consultation and also use them for teaching purposes.

3.2.7 Mental Health Issues Faced by the Community

The study showed that transgenders were at high risk of mental health problems such as depression, anxiety, and isolation because of their different gender and physical identity. They were abused physically and emotionally. They were violated by their families and by society. They often left their home at an early age.

They were abused (physically and sexually) by partners, clients, police, communities, *gurus,* and others. As far as their *gurus* were concerned, however, even if they beat and abused them, the deep emotion that they felt for them did not change.

> When our guru beats us, it feels like our father is beating us for our mistakes...we feel more like a family.

3.2.8 Motivations for Self-care

The study showed that when transgenders were unaware about the risks of unprotected sex they were at high risk of HIV and STIs (Fig. 3.3). With increased awareness in the community over time through NGOs and peers, they became more informed, aware, and concerned about their sexual and reproductive health. NGOs provided them regular medical checkups and counseling and also motivated them to follow self-care practices.

> At the end of the day, our livelihood and lives depend on our appearance and presentation. The more healthy we are, the more beautiful we will be and the more we will be desired. So, we will earn more money!

3.2.9 A Transgender's Personal Narrative on Self-care

Documented By: Dr. Rashmi Pachauri Rajan
Anchal is a transgender who has lived among the transgender community for over 25 years. Anchal always felt that she was a woman trapped in a man's body. Even as a small child, she was very effeminate and her friends, classmates, and even her teachers often commented on her effeminate mannerisms. When Anchal was in Class 5, she began to realize that she was "different," and began to perceive her feelings of effeminism more starkly—she liked to dress in girls' clothes, wear makeup, loved to dance, and perform in women's roles.

When Anchal entered high school, she got physically involved with a boy her age who had been adopted by her parents and was living with them. And around this time, she was propositioned for sex by the physical instructor at her school. It was also at around the same time that her family, particularly her mother and

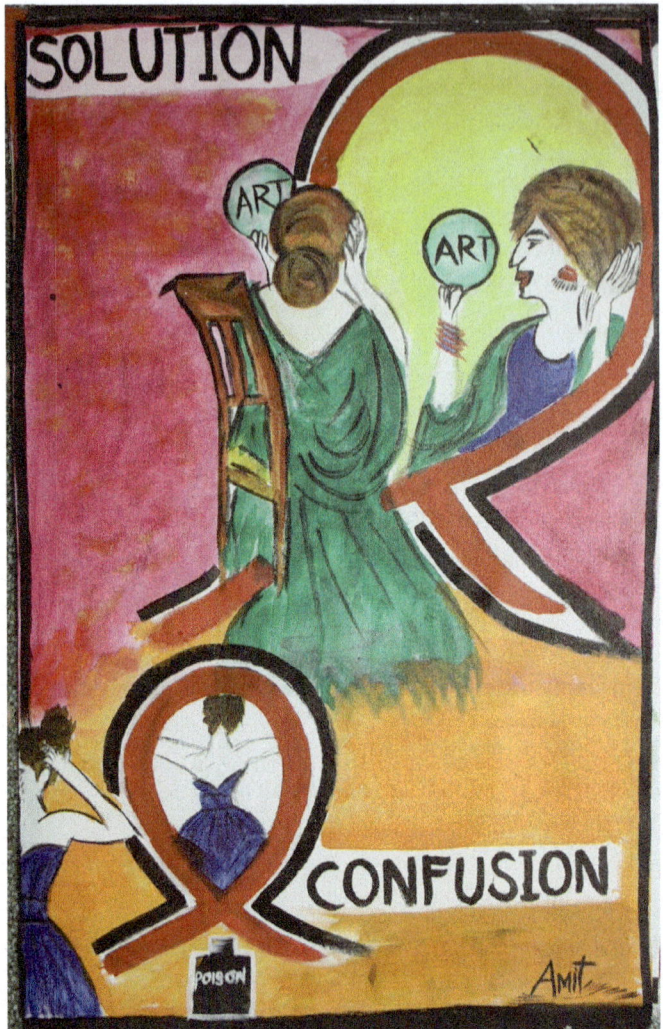

Fig. 3.3 Addressing risk painting by Amit (Sanjana)

brothers, began to notice the stark differences in her behavior as compared to that of her brothers. Anchal loved to dance and perform on stage during local festivals and special occasions, and was known for her dances and acting in women's roles. And coming from an economically relatively weak background, more and more her mother began encouraging her to perform, as it supplemented the much-needed money requirements of her family. Looking back, Anchal feels that by then most people—her family, friends, and even people in her neighborhood—knew she was transgender. But she still did not quite realize it, mainly because she was not, at that time, aware of or informed enough about what transgender really was.

However, as this realization began to dawn on Anchal gradually and she began to identify herself with the transgender community, she began to spend more and more time with them. She started living with them (and visiting her family on occasion). She began working, in the first instance, as a beggar at major road intersections and on local trains, as a lot of transgender in India do. By and by, she started doing sex work, till finally sex work, in fact, became her regular occupation.

It was about 25 years ago that Anchal got to know of and then became involved with the Humsafar Trust (HST), when the organization started in Mumbai, India. The Humsafar Trust was initially founded to reach out to LGBTQ communities in the Mumbai Metro and surrounding areas. It began with conducting workshops on issues of HIV/AIDS and human rights of LGBTQ, and it soon became evident that the trust would also have to work aggressively on the health and human rights of the community.

Anchal and her transgender friends used to come to the area where the current HST office is located, for tea and snacks at a small stall below the office building. In this process, they often met with the then staff of the organization, who would invite them into the office, chat with them informally, and, at the same time, provide them with information on HIV prevention and safe sex. Anchal subsequently started working with HST as a peer educator. She was an avid and eager learner and took to heart everything she was taught.

Between what she learned at HST and what she picked up having worked for a short while as a compounder/helper for a local doctor when she was in high school, Anchal has become extremely health and hygiene conscious. Her awareness of and information about the various aspects of self-care are high, be it related to the use of condoms, gels, or medication, including the use of antibiotics. For example, she is adamant about using condoms during her sex work, even often in the face of threats of violence from clients. She gets regular medical checks provided by various NGOs, including HST, and has HIV testing done every six months. Anchal does not consider affordability of medication or self-care products an issue. Her view on this is that "*if I am unwell and something has been prescribed by a doctor and is not available or provided by an NGO, I will buy and use it, regardless of the cost, because I consider my health and well-being of foremost importance.*"

Her self-care practices also include healthy and hygienic nutrition ("*I cook my own food and drink only boiled or bottled water*") she detoxes herself with a glass of hot water and *Chavanprash* (a well-known and popular Indian Ayurvedic tonic) every morning. She uses some of the best branded makeup products because she feels they will not harm her skin and will enhance her looks—something that is very important for her as a sex worker. She keeps herself, her clothes, and her surroundings clean and well kept, and keeps herself protected from physical harm.

Anchal realizes that in her profession as well as in her community, violence is rampant and almost a given. This violence takes the shape of physical and sexual abuse, often from within the family, client-related violence, partner violence (sexual, physical, and emotional), police violence, and sometimes violence from members of the society who view transgender as "different," lowly or frightening.

With respect to police-related violence, Anchal says it has to be "managed" in that she and other transgender within a given "territory" make themselves known to the police in that area and pay them an allotted amount per month for operating from that area. Once a mutually beneficial relationship has been established, then the police become "allies" to an extent and do not bother the community. In fact, they actively protect them at times.

Anchal is now 48 years old and is a respected "*guru*" (an influential leader or teacher among the transgender community in her locality). She treats her 16 "*chelas*" (disciples or students—who are other transgender) as her own children, looking after their needs, safety, and often even helping them financially with transitioning, if required.

Anchal herself took a decision not to transition, for a variety of reasons. She feels that, having lived among the transgender community, she knows what difficult lives they lead, more so she feels, if they have transitioned. But an even more important reason for her having decided not to transition is that she "*wants to return to God in the same form as God sent (me) to this earth.*" She visits her parents regularly, and by now they know, and even accept, that she is transgender as well as that she is a sex worker. She supports not just her parents, but even her two brothers and their families (as both her brothers are alcoholics and unemployed) financially and emotionally. But even though her parents are aware of her transgender identity, given the society they live in, their culture and conventions, they would be embarrassed and fall from grace were it publicly known that one of their sons is transgender. To keep intact her family's reputation and standing in their community, Anchal makes sure she dresses and behaves like a man when she visits them. Needless to say, this puts enormous emotional pressure on her and has, at times, led her to depression and anxiety.

Anchal has been in a long-term relationship with a man for over 20 years. For reasons beyond her control, her partner got married a few years ago. Given the strength of her relationship Anchal has with her partner, his wife and children (he has two) know about his relationship with Anchal. In fact, Anchal is accepted as part of their family and is referred to as "Big Mummy" by the children.

She is invited to attend important family functions and contributes to the family as and when required, financially and with respect to their seeking health and other advice from her on occasion. However, "*it would be a lie,*" she admits, "*if I said my boyfriend's marriage did not affect me. I went into a deep depression for weeks after it took place.*" Anchal says she did not seek counseling nor consult a doctor for her depression. Instead, she turned to religion—she spent long hours in temples and mosques, praying and introspecting. And her "*chelas*" who care about her deeply helped enormously to get her out of her depression. This is strong evidence of self-help—in the form of social support systems from within the community! Another example of mental health self-care that Anchal discussed (though she admits she has not yet participated in nor initiated this among her community) is the formation of a WhatsApp (or other suchlike) group of like-minded and similar people (in this case, members of the transgender community who are there for each other as and when needed or in times of crises). Anchal admits that she consumes alcohol everyday ("*I take no more than two drinks ever*"), but says she has never smoked nor taken recreational drugs, as those, she feels, are harmful to health. The one thing that Anchal included in her self-care practices is a life insurance policy, which she says is very important for a person like her, if ever the need for it arose. It keeps her secure and ensures that she will not have to depend on anyone if she were to get sick or, even after her death, to take care of her funeral. It will also take care of her family after she is no more.

Anchal's self-care quotient is very high, especially given her background, education (she is a Class 10 passed student), and that she is transgender. She believes, "*If one takes care of oneself, then that will automatically lead to good health, which will result in happiness. Life is precious and beautiful and should be thus valued. And for us, because our earnings depend on how we look and present ourselves, health is everything. One should strive to be a role model for others, no matter what walk of life one comes from.*"

3.3 Discussion

Sexuality was once considered an unimportant issue in the Indian social sphere. But now it is vibrant and political. There is a fight for the legal and social rights of lesbians, gays, bisexuals, and transgender which is supported by healthcare NGOs, human rights activists, and feminists. Together, they form contemporary India's queer movement. Once a derogatory word, today queer is accepted as an identity signifying a sexual orientation.

Transgender experience their identity in a variety of ways and may become aware of their transgender identity at any age. Some can trace their transgender identity and feelings back to their earliest memories. They may have vague feelings of "not fitting in" with people of their assigned sex. Others become aware of their transgender identities or begin to explore and experience gender non-conforming attitudes and behaviors during adolescence or much later in life. Some embrace their transgender feelings, while others struggle with feelings of shame or confusion. Those who transitioned later in life may have struggled to fit in adequately with their assigned sex only to later face dissatisfaction with their lives. Some transgenders, transsexuals in particular, experience intense dissatisfaction with their sex assigned at birth, physical sex characteristics, or the gender role associated with that sex. These individuals often seek gender-affirming treatments.

Transgender usually live or prefer to live in the gender role different to the one they are assigned at birth. The preferred gender role may or may not be related to their sexual preferences. Transgender is an umbrella term that includes transsexuals, cross-dressers, intersexed persons, and gender-variant persons. Transgender can be "male-to-female" (MtF) or "female-to-male" (FtM), and sometimes referred to as "transgender woman/transwoman" and "transgender man/transman," respectively.

The term used for transgender in India is *hijra*. An older name for *hijras* is *kinnar*, which is used by some *hijra* groups as a more respectable and formal term.

An abusive slang for *hijra* in Hindi is *chakka* [13]. *Hijras* in Tamil Nadu identify as "*aravani.*" Tamil Nadu Aravanigal Welfare Board, a state government initiative under the Department of Social Welfare, defines *aravanis* as biological males who self-identity themselves as a woman trapped in a male body. Some *aravanis* want the public and media to use the term "*thirunangi*" [13]. Globally, transgenders are referred to as the third gender.

Hijras make their presence felt at marriages and births where they bestow their blessings. They are, however, a highly stigmatized community. *Hijras* usually live in large communities. The head of such a community is the *guru*. This community has a hierarchical *guru–shishya* (teacher–disciple) structure and exists as a parallel society within the existing Indian culture [14–16]. The *akwa hijras* are not yet castrated but are in preparation for castration after specific rites. These *hijras* are males who cross-dress or wear female attire (*khada-kothis*) and have joined *hijra gharanas* (adopted families) after leaving their biological families. The *nirvaan hijras* are ritually castrated men who are a part of ritual housing called *gharanas*. *Jogtas* are Hindu *hijras* who are male temple prostitutes [17].

However, with increased urbanization and changing societal structures in India, the traditional roles of these transgender have lost their importance. Consequently, many of the male-to-female transgender have become sex workers, particularly in urban centers such as Mumbai. They experience a high prevalence of STIs including HIV and have significantly higher number of sex partners [14]. Their health-seeking behaviors are often limited due to stigmatization in healthcare settings [15].

Health Problems

A transgender health assessment should involve recognition of possible gender identity disorder, history-taking with respect to prior and current use of hormones or surgical interventions, as well as general physical, mental, and sexual health histories. Physical and screening tests need to be based on the organ systems present rather than the perceived gender of the patient. Physicians should be aware of common hormone regimens and their associated risks. Finally, patients can best explore transgender issues in a setting of respect and trust in which confidentiality concerns are addressed, and clinic staff are educated about transgender issues [16].

The link between mental health disorders and discrimination has been established. The coming-out process for an older LGBT person, who has lived most of his or her life in a hostile or intolerant environment, can induce significant stress and contribute to lower life satisfaction and self-esteem. Managing social stressors such as prejudice, stigmatization, violence, and internalized homophobia over long periods of time results in higher risk of depression, suicide, risky behavior, and substance abuse. LGBT populations, therefore, may be at increased risk for these and other mental disorders. There is a high lifetime prevalence of mental disorders in LGBT persons [18,19].

3.3 Discussion

Education, Employment, and Legal Rights

In India, most transgenders have little or no education. Consequently, they are usually not formally employed and are often forced into sex work and begging. On April 2014, the Supreme Court of India passed a landmark judgment reaffirming individuals' right to choose their identity, as male, female, or third gender. The Supreme Court judgment which cites a UNDP India study in its verdict also instructed central and state governments to develop inclusive social welfare schemes and ensure greater involvement of the transgender community in policy formulation [20].

In India, *hijras* now have the option to identify as a eunuch ("E") on passports and on certain government documents. The Election Commission forms now have a separate column "O" for "others" (transgender or *hijras*) in the voter enrollment and registration forms. Following in the footsteps of the Election Commission, the Unique Identification Authority of India (UIDAI) also recognizes transgender. Enrollment forms of the UIDAI have a third column of "T" for "Transgender" along with "M" and "F" for "Male" and "Female," respectively [21].

Self-care among transgender has an important place in improving their health and their lives. Self-care is practiced by many transgenders, but there is considerable scope for improvement. Research is needed to assess how and in which areas self-care can be enhanced to improve the lives of transgender. Growing access to the Internet has facilitated the process of increasing self-care to improve the health and well-being of transgender.

References

1. Hirschfeld M, Cauldwell. Negotiating the borders of the gender regime. Federal Republic of Germany. 1923.
2. Prince VC. Men who choose to be women. Sexology. 1969 February.
3. Elkins R. Sex as a biological or physiological quality. MediLexicon International. 1985.
4. Swanstrom NA. Developing and implementing a scale to assess attitudes regarding transsexuality. Carolina Arts. 2014 February; 18(2).
5. World Health Organization. WHO consolidated guideline on self-care interventions for health: Sexual and reproductive health and rights. Geneva: World Health Organization; 2019.
6. Herbst JH, Jacobs ED, Finlayson TJ, McKleroy VS, Neumann MS, Crepaz N. Estimating HIV prevalence and risk behaviors of transgender persons in the United States: A systematic review. AIDS Behav. 2008;12(1):1–17.
7. Stroumsa D. The state of transgender health care: Policy, law, and medical frameworks. Am J Public Health. 2014;104(3):31–8.
8. Victoria M. Integrative women's health. American Psychiatric Association. 2013;745.
9. Chisolm-Straker M, Jardine L, Bennouna C, Morency-Brassard N, Coy L, Egemba MO, Shearer PL. Transgender and gender nonconforming in emergency departments: A qualitative report of patient experiences. Mary Ann Liebert, Inc. 2017;2(1):8–16.
10. Gay and Lesbian Alliance against Defamation. GLAAD, USA; 2011 February 4.
11. Bradford, Judith, Reisner, Sari L, Honnold, Julie A, Xavier, Jessica. Experiences of transgender- related discrimination and implications for health: Results from the Virginia transgender health initiative study. Am J Public Health. 2013 October;103(10):1820–29.

12. Lombardi EL, Wilchins A, Riki P, Dana MD. Gender violence: Transgender experiences with violence and discrimination. J Homosex. 2008;42(1):89–101.
13. Mal S. Let us to live: Social exclusion of hijra community. Asian J Res Soc Sci Hum. 2015;1(5):108–17.
14. Kumta S, Laurie M, Weitzen S, Jerajani H, Gogate A, Row-Kavi A, Anand V. Socio-demographic, sexual risk behavior and HIV among men who have sex with men attending voluntary counseling and testing services in Mumbai, India. Paper presented at the XV International AIDS Conference, Toronto, Canada; 2006 August.
15. Deshmukh V, Row Kavi A, Anand V. Stigmatization of transgender individuals: A barrier to access of health services. Paper presented at the XV International Conference on AIDS, Bangkok, Thailand; 2004 July.
16. Feldman J, Bockting W. Transgender health: Transgender persons represent an underserved community in need of sensitive, comprehensive healthcare. Minnesota Medical. 2003;86(7):25–32.
17. Robertson J. MSM Circle: Empowering communities of men who have sex with men to prevent HIV. Humsafar Trust, Mumbai; 2008.
18. Brotman S, Ryan B, Cormier R. The health and social service needs of gay and lesbian elders and their families in Canada. Gerontologist. 2003;43(2):192–202.
19. Dean L, Med, Meyer IH, Robinson K, Sell R, Scd, Sember R, Silenzio VMB, Bowen DJ, Bradford JB, Rothblum E, White J, Dunn P, Lawrence A, Wolf D, Xavier J, Carter D, Pittman J, Tierney R. Lesbian, gay, bisexual, and transgender health: Findings and concerns. J Gay Lesbian Med Assoc. 2000 Sep.
20. United Nations Development Programme. A development agenda for transgenders in Maharashtra. United Nations Development Programme.
21. Sinha S. Social exclusion of transgender in the civil society: A case study of the status of the transgender in Kolkata. Int J Humanit Soc Sci Stud. 2016;3(2):178–90.
22. Bakshi S. A comparative analysis of hijras and drag queens: The subversive possibilities and limits of parading effeminacy and negotiating masculinity. J Homosex. 2005;46:211–23.
23. Nanda S. The hijras of India: Cultural and individual dimensions of an institutionalized third gender role. J Homosex. 1985;11(3–4):35–54.
24. Shreedhar, J. HIV thrives in ancient traditions. Harv AIDS Rev. 1995;10–1.

Open Access This chapter is licensed under the terms of the Creative Commons Attribution 4.0 International License (http://creativecommons.org/licenses/by/4.0/), which permits use, sharing, adaptation, distribution and reproduction in any medium or format, as long as you give appropriate credit to the original author(s) and the source, provide a link to the Creative Commons license and indicate if changes were made.

The images or other third party material in this chapter are included in the chapter's Creative Commons license, unless indicated otherwise in a credit line to the material. If material is not included in the chapter's Creative Commons license and your intended use is not permitted by statutory regulation or exceeds the permitted use, you will need to obtain permission directly from the copyright holder.

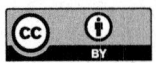

Chapter 4
Female Sex Work Dynamics: Empowerment, Mobilization, Mobility

4.1 Backdrop

UNAIDS defines sex work as selling sexual services [1]. Sex workers involved in sexual relations with multiple partners are a key group of women who need access to comprehensive sexual health services, including HIV prevention, treatment, and care [2]. There are a broad range of sex workers in various locations including those who are street-based and brothel-based, those who work as escorts, and those who work from their own homes. Some women exchange sex for cash or goods but do not see themselves as sex workers [3–5]. Migrant sex workers are particularly at high risk of HIV [6]. Globally, female sex workers are 13.5% more likely to be living with HIV than other women of reproductive age [7]. In Asia, female sex workers are almost 30% more likely to be living with HIV than other women. Unprotected sex with multiple partners puts sex workers at high risk of HIV [8]. In India, targeted HIV interventions for female sex workers are found to be highly cost-effective [9]. However, interventions must be adapted to meet the needs of sex workers in different settings.

To address structural barriers and ensure human rights, WHO supports countries to implement a comprehensive package of HIV and health services for sex workers through community-led approaches [7]. Programs that enhance sex workers' ability to use condoms are also vitally important [2, 10]. Health interventions for prevention of sexual transmission of HIV and other STIs among sex workers include condom programming, harm reduction interventions for those who inject drugs, behavioral interventions, HIV testing and counseling, HIV treatment and care, pre-exposure prophylaxis (PrEP), prevention and management of viral hepatitis, tuberculosis, mental health conditions, and sexual and reproductive health problems.

Lack of safe and supportive working conditions and violation of human rights render sex workers vulnerable to HIV infection through actions such as confiscating condoms, using condoms as evidence against sex workers and violence against sex workers. Female sex workers have difficulty in accessing health services in many parts of the world due to criminalization of sex work. Because of criminalization, sex workers are less able to negotiate condom use and are subjected to violence by clients [11]. Globally, decriminalization of sex work could lead to a 46% reduction in new HIV infections in sex workers and eliminating sexual violence against sex workers could lead to a 20% reduction in new HIV infections [12].

Sex workers have basic human rights to prevention, care, and treatment [13]. Most interventions currently focus on prevention and condom use. Sex workers should also have equitable access to antiretroviral therapy. In many countries, such as India, no published data are available on the number of sex workers receiving antiretroviral therapy [14]. As a vulnerable population, it is very critical for sex workers with HIV to have access to treatment [15]. There is, however, an increase in the number of sex workers accessing antiretroviral therapy with the help of peer educators, as well as trained, non-judgmental providers [14].

Legal frameworks are needed to protect human rights. There should be mandatory measures by governments such as compulsory HIV testing of sex workers. Interventions that improve HIV knowledge and protective behaviors, particularly condom use, as well as those that respect human rights are the key to successfully preventing HIV among female sex workers.

In addition to legal reform, programs that take an empowerment approach, such as the Sonagachi Project and Sagram in India, have shown to create better working conditions and have been most effective in reducing HIV acquisition by female sex workers [16, 17]. Female sex workers themselves have led some of the most effective, evidence-based responses [18]. Empowering female sex workers with the means to protect themselves has worked effectively for HIV prevention.

4.2 Research on Female Sex Workers

Research was undertaken to study the values, preferences, and practices with regard to self-care for sexual and reproductive health and rights (SRHR) and HIV prevention and treatment in female sex workers. The objectives were to obtain an understanding of their views about self-care practices; how they obtained information on self-care interventions; what were their motivations to use them; what barriers they faced while using them; and what they did if self-care practices failed.

Research was undertaken in Delhi and Tamil Nadu. A qualitative study design was employed. In-depth interviews (IDIs), focus group discussions (FGDs), key informant interviews (KIIs), and a workshop were conducted with female sex workers. Qualitative research methods allowed greater spontaneity and interaction with participants. They provided an opportunity to the participants to respond elaborately and in greater detail. The interviews were conducted using interview guides. The interviews were approximately 90–120 minutes in length. The interviews were recorded, and the recordings were transcribed and checked for accuracy. Two IDIs, two KIIs, and one FGD (8–10 participants) were conducted in Delhi.

One workshop was conducted in Tamil Nadu with 15 female sex workers who were HIV positive to understand their general health problems, sexual health and HIV issues, and how they accessed information on SRH products and services on social media and other platforms.

For the key informant interviews, participants were selected on the basis of their experience. They were peer educators working with NGOs. For in-depth interviews, outreach workers with 4–5 years of experience were selected. Focus group discussions included peer educators, outreach workers, and other young female sex workers. During the workshop, participants were asked to depict their sexual practices in art form for which they were provided with colors and canvas.

Triangulation of data generated by KIIs, IDIs, FGDs, and the workshop made it possible to obtain reliable information on complex issues. Ethical approval for undertaking the study was granted by the Ethical Review Board of the Humsafar Trust. Before initiating the study, participants were given consent forms which described the study. Consent of all participants was taken in writing and orally. Confidentiality of all participants was assured.

4.2.1 Research Findings

The findings include a discussion of the feelings and behaviors of female sex workers; self-care interventions for SRHR; information sources for SRHR; risks and barriers faced by the community; and motivations for self-care.

4.2.2 Involvement in Sex Work

Study participants including sex workers, peer educators, healthcare providers, and counselors indicated that social exclusion due to poverty, low income, unemployment, lack of education, little or no social support from the family, and adverse living conditions dragged women into sex work.

Because they were not qualified to get well-paid jobs and were harassed by their employers at their workplace, women engaged in sex work. They disliked their work and found that sex work was their best or only option to make a living. Some were agnostic about sex work but found that it offered flexibility and good pay.

> The conditions of our workplace were harassing, there was no flexibility in working hours, and sex work offers us a better pay off.

Generally, migrants from poor regions who were unable to find work to meet their basic needs ended up in the sex work industry.

> In order to earn our livelihood, we prefer to get involved in sex work; this is the easiest way for us.

Sex workers, like most workers, had diverse feelings about their work.

> We enjoy our work and find it rewarding and fun which is not so with other work.

4.2.3 Self-care Interventions for Health and Family Planning

The study showed that for common conditions, such as fever and flu, sex workers first tried homemade, herbal remedies. If they did not work, or they still needed help, then they visited the pharmacy (preferably the one that they accessed regularly). If they still needed help, they visited a health clinic. For HIV and sexually transmitted infections (STIs), they usually visited a health provider at a non-governmental organization (NGO) usually one that they regularly associated with. Only when absolutely necessary, they visited health centers, mostly government-run health centers.

> We visit clinics in severe conditions only, else we prefer home-made remedies.

Female sex workers preferred to use condoms as they could get them free of cost from NGOs or their clients brought them. The use of creams and gels among female sex workers was rare as the NGOs did not provide these and they had to purchase these products from medical stores.

> We only use condoms as contraceptives. Creams and gels are difficult for us to buy.

The study indicates that consistent use of condoms was difficult with partners who refused to use condoms and promised to pay more instead. Sometimes, for fear of losing their clients, they did not insist on using condoms.

> We easily get ready for sexual encounters without protection to retain our clients.

Female sex workers faced the risk of unwanted pregnancy and sexually transmitted diseases (Fig. 4.1). They had unmet needs for contraceptives and required more comprehensive interventions for sexually and reproductive health (SRH).

> As we agree to have sex without condoms; we face the risk of pregnancy and have to get aborted.

Female sex workers were informed about modern contraceptives by the peer educators of the NGOs but had limited access to them. The study shows that because of lack of social support, limited resources, fear of violence from the clients, poverty, and unemployment, female sex workers compromised their own health and well-being.

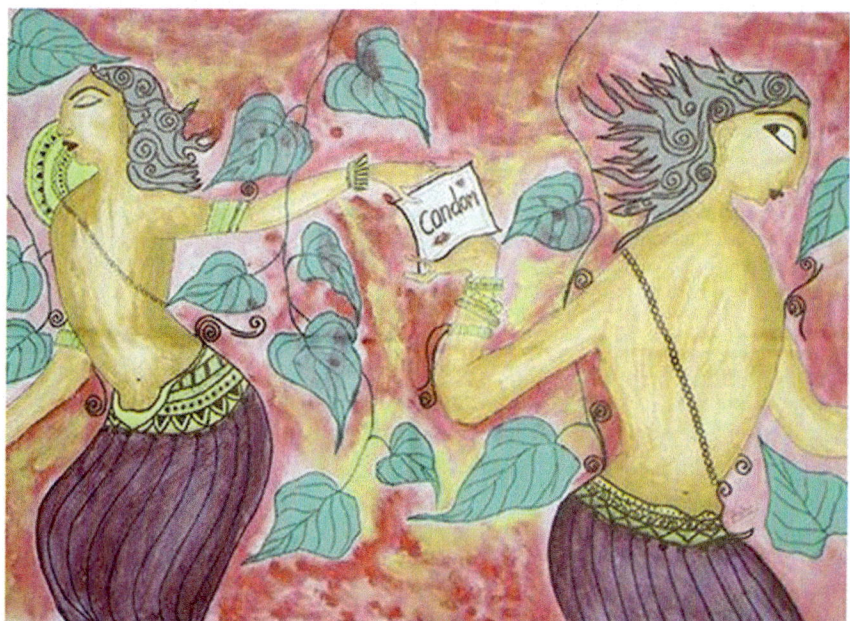

Fig. 4.1 Female sex workers access condoms painting by Ashu (Bips)

4.2.4 Information Sources

Data on sex workers in different places revealed that it was important for women who trade sex for money, to have knowledge about HIV prevention and sexual and reproductive health. Female sex workers got information through social media, mass media, and their interpersonal contacts, i.e., peer educators and outreach workers. Through television and radio, they got information related to condom use for safe sex. The study findings suggest that women who were involved in sex work generally got information from NGOs and outreach workers. NGO workers undertook behavior change communication programs to make them more aware about sexual and reproductive health. NGOs conducted condom demonstrations and also provided information on hygienic practices that female sex workers should follow.

Female sex workers generally obtained products such as antibiotics, condoms, creams, and gels from NGOs who also provided regular checkups for detection of syphilis and HIV testing. Thus, NGOs provided female sex workers services and also informed them about safe and protected sex.

> I use condoms. NGO told me to use these. They taught me how to use a condom when I joined there. When I first went there, they asked me to take an HIV test and I refused, but they made me understand that this was for my own benefit.

4.2.5 Risks and Barriers Faced by the Community

Women traded sex for money because they faced poverty issues. They lacked support from their families. When they had children, they had to bring them up alone.

> We are all alone to look after our children and our families. Our parents do not support us. Our husbands also rely on us for their extravagant lifestyles. They indulge in debauchery. We have no option except to trade sex for our livelihood. Some of us are forcefully thrown into the sex trade by our husbands.

The study shows that because female sex workers were stigmatized by the health system, they were afraid to visit doctors. When they had a problem, they preferred to take medicines from the pharmacies. However, if they were unable to explain their problems related to sexual health to the pharmacist, they could take the wrong medicine which resulted in harmful effects.

> We have a fear of breach of confidentiality, and so we avoid visiting the healthcare facilities.

4.2.6 Mental Health Problems Faced by the Community

Women in sex work traded sex for money; their sexual encounters generally involved sex without any emotional attachment. The study reveals that these women faced mental health problems and were ill-treated and abused by the community, police, and others (Fig. 4.2).

> We are sexually abused by the police and other men around us. They do not pay us after sexual intercourse and sometimes they bring 4–5 men with them to abuse us.

They faced stigma in society which resulted in mental depression and isolation. They actively chose sex work because they found more perks in sex work than in other jobs.

> If we have to get abused anyway, we might as well earn through sex work.

4.2.7 Violence Faced by the Community

The study shows that female sex workers experienced physical, psychological as well as sexual violence by the community. They were forced to have sex with men in their own families. They were threatened and abused by their family. They were also beaten up by the older members of their families.

4.2 Research on Female Sex Workers

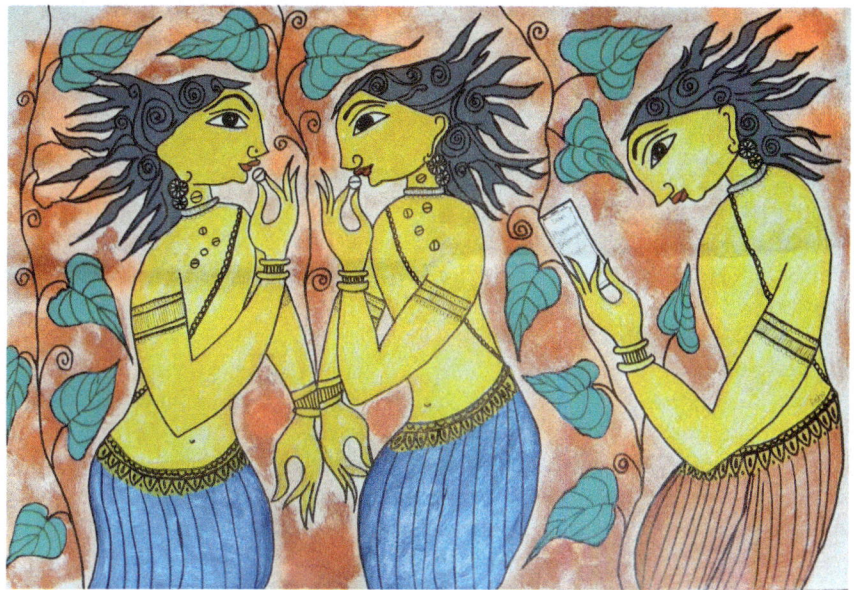

Fig. 4.2 Female sex workers seek protection painting by Ashu (Bips)

We are humiliated and threatened by our families and fear the loss of custody of our children.

They were abused sexually and were denied their basic rights. They were forced to consume alcohol and drugs and were sometimes arrested by the police for carrying condoms. Female sex workers also faced verbal abuse because customers and other community members saw them as undesirable women in the society.

People call us 'whore' and bully us.

4.2.8 Motivation for Self-care

The study shows that when female sex workers were not aware about HIV and other sexually transmitted diseases, they frequently had sex without protection. At times, their clients forced them to have sex without protection by bribing them with extra money. Through their association with NGOs, they become more informed about sexual and reproductive health. Consequently, they refused to have sex without protection even if they were offered more money. With increasing awareness through different programs, female sex workers become more concerned about their sexual and reproductive health. They got motivated to use self-care through workshops organized by NGOs to enhance their awareness of the importance of following self-care practices.

4.2.9 A Female Sex Worker with AIDS: Personal Narrative on Self-care

Documented By: Philo Magadalene A.

Women driven to sex work face intersectional oppression encountering the very realities that they seek to overcome. As they struggle to confront, cope with, and survive these conditions, it is only normal that self-care tends to take a backseat.

This is the story of an HIV-positive widow who turned to sex work out of sheer desperation to feed the family, and whose self-care practices were purely driven by the motive that she, being the only breadwinner of the family, could not let her children be orphaned.

Vijaya along with her one-year-old daughter was diagnosed with HIV in the year 1998. Having received the infection from her alcoholic husband who had an illegitimate affair, Vijaya did not know that he had been infected until then. She shuddered when the nurse said, "*You have AIDS. You will die in four years. You already have two daughters with you. Get them married soon.*" AIDS had been the go-to word as nobody used the term "HIV" then. Having been abandoned by her second husband and left alone to fend for the family of four children, she sunk further into poverty with heightened vulnerabilities. Her health conditions did not allow her to be a domestic helper anymore. She realized, "*How will people in the houses accept me for work if I keep scratching myself?*" Sex work appeared to be the only plausible option.

Vijaya's knowledge about sexual and reproductive health was limited before she entered sex work. But she knew well enough to visit the medical health facility when she needed anything. That was how she aborted her fourth child who was conceived soon after the delivery of the younger child. When she conceived again for the last time, she resorted to unsafe abortion through hearsay remedies like papaya, sesame, and palm sugar, but had to reach out to the government hospital after three months when nothing worked. By then, it was too late for safe abortion. She pleasantly recalls, "*I was told, 'Be it a boy or a girl, give birth and raise the child.' Now that is the daughter who is feeding me.*" Vijaya underwent family planning surgery 14 days after her fourth child was born.

Vijaya's first experience with sex work was at a prostitution home she used to visit. Since her knowledge about condoms and safe sex practices came only from interaction with non-governmental organizations (NGOs), one can believe that before this relationship with NGOs, she was involved in high-risk sexual behaviors during her time in the prostitution home. In addition to health vulnerabilities, she also put herself at social risk. She remembers a time when her landlord visited the prostitution home as a client and she had to request someone else to attend to him because she "*didn't want him knocking at my door in the middle of the night causing problems.*" At this point in Vijaya's life, one sees no instance of positive self-care behavior in terms of sexual and reproductive health.

Realizing the dangers that come with visiting a prostitution home, Vijaya decided to stop going there and began attending to clients in their own homes or in her home. As she went to the District Collectorate every morning in search of customers, she got introduced to NGOs like Teddy, Russ Foundation, and Thaai Vizhudhugal who looked out for people like her in that place. A person from an NGO told her, "*There are so many NGOs. Just by attending all their meetings, you can get around 600 per month.*" In pursuit of an alternate way to earn, Vijaya promptly made use of this opportunity and began attending different NGO meetings in exchange for food and money. Despite this motive, she did end up receiving crucial learnings about self-care that were of much higher value.

Vijaya learned about the importance of condoms and regularly received a sufficient number of these from the NGOs. She says, "*There are places in bus stands, where you can place the money and get condoms. I never take from there because I always have what the NGO gives me.*" After she learned about the indispensable nature of condoms, she began carrying one in her handbag wrapped in a newspaper always and strictly ensured that the customers used it. Usage of condoms was one continuous self-care routine that she practiced because she believed this: "*I don't want them to face what I am going through by living with HIV.*" Even for a self-care routine as simple as the usage of condoms, Vijaya faced several barriers. Many clients, assuming that "*Free condoms won't be good*" or that "*they will break,*" refused to use the condom she offered. Speaking of this difficulty, she admits, "*I won't tell them that I am infected. If they know that, they won't come to me.*"

The condom was not the only contraceptive that the NGOs introduced to Vijaya and her community members. Speaking of an instance when an NGO proposed the use of female condoms and offered them samples, Vijaya says, "*I didn't like it. But some people did, because, with female condoms, they could attend to their clients without any issues even when they were having their periods.*"

In addition to the quality information provided by NGOs, Vijaya also acted on the information she received from pharmacies. More often than not, the medicines she took were to ensure that she could continue her work without any hindrance. She made frequent visits to the pharmacy requesting medicines that would postpone her period because she had to "*visit the temple.*" Her ignorance and lack of knowledge about such health practices led to complications that Vijaya never anticipated. When she turned 40, she began having intense flow lasting for 15–20 days that no amount of medications could control. The government hospital refused to operate on her, and the private facility was too expensive for her to afford. She blames herself for the situation she was in saying, "*I didn't know we were not supposed to take that tablet a lot.*" Only after she produced a letter from an influential activist did the government hospital decide to treat her.

Vijaya's dependence on the pharmacy was not restricted to period delay medicines alone. She dealt with the frequent STIs by approaching the pharmacy and buying tablets for amounts as little as 15 rupees. At times when that did not work, she visited the government hospital receiving a prescription for 15 days which she would reuse the next time she had the same infection. Vijaya's reliance on medicines dispensed in the pharmacy may be seen as a form of a self-care routine, but it also points to her high-risk behavior. Through pharmacies, she had open access to an excess amount of medicines like Brufen and Paracetamol that she had little knowledge about. She says, *"For a long time, I had thought I could take as much Paracetamol as I wanted because it won't affect my body."*

One can understand that the self-care that Vijaya believed in practicing to manage her health issues was partly driven by faulty assumptions and myths. Having been sensitized by the NGOs about the importance of condoms, she moved with the belief that condoms are enough to protect oneself and maintain good sexual and reproductive health. Once, when the doctors strictly insisted that she limits the number of clients and avoids excessive use of tablets to deal with the recurring sores in her vagina, she argued that *"the customers are using condoms anyway."* She only realized she was wrong when they told her, *"this has nothing to do with that."*

Given her illiteracy and poverty, the only sources she could count on for health-related information were NGOs, pharmacies, and government health facilities. Vijaya's account of doctors in the government hospital reveals that she received constant lectures from them advising her to *"exercise self-control," "go for construction labor,"* and not *"make your child an orphan,"* It sometimes even went to the extent of making her cry. The doctors insisted that she should come to the hospital for any ailment instead of visiting the pharmacy. But, interestingly, one notices that the support Vijaya received in terms of knowledge and information was much better from the pharmacy. For example, when Vijaya wanted to know about a particular injection she received in the hospital, the doctor had said, *"Even if I tell you, are you going to understand?"* But whenever she asked from the pharmacy what a particular tablet was for, they said, *"It's for pain. Don't take it too much. If you take too much, it'll affect your kidney."* Or when she asked for *"three strips of painkillers,"* they advised her to *"take one, as and when it was really necessary."* Although it is not appropriate for a pharmacist to take over the duty of the doctor, when it came to informing and sensitizing the patient, in Vijaya's case, it was the pharmacy that usually provided her the support she needed.

NGOs were Vijaya's monumental support system attempting to address her intersectional vulnerabilities. They played a critical role in ensuring that condom usage and other positive health behaviors become a part of Vijaya's self-care routine and that she understood the importance of her medications for HIV. She notes, *"They tell me that even if I had nothing to eat, I must at least have a biscuit and tea and take my medications, and at no cost, should I stop my medication."* Aside from sensitizing people, NGOs also provided emotional support whenever Vijaya needed it. It was a space she could impulsively reach out to anytime she needed anything.

Vijaya's strong dependence on NGOs can be explained by the fact that she lacked social support elsewhere. With her parents and even some of her children not knowing about her HIV status and sex work, Vijaya did not have anybody to confide things. She was not closely involved with her peers preferring to keep her affairs to herself. Her discretion stemmed from many obvious reasons. Vijaya was especially wary of her neighbors finding out about her situation and creating problems. She says, *"They used to ask, 'Why do you always go to the government hospital and get medicines? What medicine is that? What is it for?'... If I had told them the truth, they wouldn't have let me stay."* Many years back, when the school her daughter studied in discovered the child's positive status, they made her sit outside in the rain during examinations because she had gotten sick. Vijaya fought with the teachers and removed her from that school the same day.

Besides these social struggles, the financial burdens she had to wade through to make ends meet only enhanced her vulnerability. A customer of hers intermittently lived with her offering to support the family, but it was not enough for her to quit her work. She borrowed from neighbors and local rowdies owing them a large amount of money that grew with cumulative interests daily. There were times when she had to lock the door from the outside and stay inside with her children or vacate the house abandoning everything in the wee hours of the morning.

Having quit sex work for three years now, she currently lives in a government-sanctioned house, having neighbors who have lived through similar experiences like her.

Speaking of self-care, Vijaya says, *"Self-care to me is, taking good care of my own body—not attending to more customers than my body can handle and immediately visiting the doctor at the hospital if I have any ailments. If it is just a headache or fever, I'll be all right by just tablets, but if I have any other problems I will cancel everything I have to do and run to the hospital first thing in the morning. One must take care of oneself in such a way that one doesn't have any ailments."*

Like all breadwinners of a family, her motive for self-care stems from the need to be alive and active for the sake of providing for her children.

4.3 Discussion

Recent estimates suggest there are approximately 8,68,000 women in India who are currently engaged in sex work [19]. Sex work is closely linked to caste discrimination, poverty, and gender inequality that is pervasive in India, with practices of underage marriage and dedication of young girls into sex work as part of religious traditions including the *"devadasi"* system in northern parts of Karnataka [20]. Although the *devadasi* system was made illegal in 1988, it is still one of the most common forms of traditional sex work in north Karnataka [21]. More than 90% of female sex workers in northern Karnataka come from *devadasi* families and represent the most marginalized "Scheduled" Castes or tribes [20].

Female sex workers have been historically blamed for the spread of STIs. In recent years, they have been held responsible for the spread of HIV [22–25]. Programs have targeted female sex workers for HIV/STI prevention [22]. While this has benefitted them, it has unfortunately increased stigma and discrimination for female sex workers as they have been labeled as "vectors of disease" [26].

Female sex workers face multiple, complex, and interdependent health problems. One example is violence which is widespread originating from a range of perpetrators including intimate partners, police, pimps, and paying partners [27, 28]. There is a growing body of evidence to show that exposure to violence among female sex workers is associated with many adverse health outcomes including: increased prevalence of HIV and sexually transmitted infections; poor emotional health; increased alcohol or drug misuse; and reduced access to STI/HIV clinics [29–32].

The mechanisms through which violence adversely affects women's health are complex and bidirectional. Violence may increase the risk of HIV/STI transmission directly through forced unprotected sex. Evidence suggests that coerced sex is rarely protected and can result in injuries that increase the risk of transmission of STIs and HIV [33–35]. Exposure to violence can also lead to depression and low self-esteem, which in turn may lead to alcohol or drug use and reduced ability to negotiate condom use. This, in turn, can compound low self-esteem and emotional health problems [36]. Additionally, broader gender inequalities that are key determinants of both STI/HIV transmission and violence among female sex workers often play an important role in reproducing gender inequalities leading to higher risk of HIV/STI transmission [37, 38]. Gender inequalities that give men power over women increase the risk of violence against women, by reducing their ability to negotiate safe and consensual sex, and hindering women's recourse to justice and help [39]. Research shows that men who are violent are more likely to have multiple concurrent partners, use condoms less frequently, have unprotected anal sex, and report substance use [40]. All these factors have been linked to increased risk of HIV/STI transmission among female sex workers [41, 42].

A significant intervention project, the Sonagachi Project (Durbar) in Kolkata, West Bengal, serves over 65,000 female sex workers annually [26, 43, 44]. The strategy employed by the Durbar project for female sex workers and their partners is to ensure consistent condom use (CCU) in every sexual encounter. A study conducted in Kolkata showed that nearly half of the female sex workers reported symptoms of STIs that required treatment in the previous 12 months [43]. It also showed that 92% of female sex workers used condoms for the prevention of pregnancy [45]. In this project, female sex workers are empowered to use condoms in every sexual encounter. Condom use is prioritized in this community because other strategies for decreasing infection such as reducing the number of sexual partners are not feasible given female sex workers' financial needs.

Female sex workers in Durbar are empowered to demand condom use by their partners. The project promotes community mobilization and condom distribution which are supported by brothel owners and peers [44, 46]. Since risk perception depends on the intimacy gradient, female sex workers may not use condoms with intimate clients and husbands [47, 48]. This may also happen if they are offered more money [49]. Newer methods such as pre-exposure prophylaxis (PrEP) are not as yet widely available to female sex workers and have not shown the same community-level impact as constant condom use [50]. Female sex workers have multiple partners whose risk behaviors outside the brothel are not known [51].

The belief that condoms decrease emotional and sexual intimacy results in condomless sexual encounters which increase the transmission of HIV/STIs

4.3 Discussion

[52–54]. Programming should, therefore, take cognizance of these factors, and strategies should be tailored to the specific needs of female sex workers and their intimate partners to prevent infection. The Sonagachi Project incorporates multiple interventions at multiple levels by including advocacy, community mobilization, micro-banking, and health services [55–57].

Over the years, it has been recognized that HIV prevention requires structural interventions to address the vulnerabilities of sex workers, including legal, physical, social, and economic factors [58–60]. UNAIDS guidelines emphasize that human rights-based approaches are the standard for HIV prevention interventions, noting that the most successful interventions occur when "female sex workers are able to assert control over their working environments, negotiate and insist on safer sex" [61]. Community mobilization is an intervention strategy that encourages collectivization to bring about structural change [59]. Community mobilization not only aims to empower marginalized key populations (particularly female sex workers) as a group for vulnerability reduction, but also increasingly allows them to make decisions and shape their own lives, which in turn influences the adoption and maintenance of low-risk behaviors [62–64]. Community-led interventions seek to change social and political structures by organizing female sex workers to confront structural barriers at multiple levels, resulting in both individual and collective empowerment [65]. The Sonagachi Project, a community mobilization project with a secondary impact on economic strengthening, is one of the best-known female sex worker interventions. It is cited as an example of a best practice and a designated HIV prevention model by the World Health Organization [43]. Inspired by the Sonagachi Project, Avahan India AIDS Initiative program is also known for its combination approach to HIV prevention that includes facilitating structural change through community mobilization.

Migration for sex work is one of the key socio-demographic drivers of the geographical spread of HIV from high- to low-HIV prevalence areas [66]. Migration is consistently reported as a potential driver of the HIV epidemic and migrants (both male and female) are at increased risk of HIV infection [67–72]. "Mobility," in terms of short-term movements, is also a crucial factor that increases the spread of HIV infection due to the higher incidence of unsafe sex along the routes of migration [73]. In India, most studies related to mobility and migration have focused on employment-related male mobility. Male mobility functions as a potential bridge for the transmission of HIV infection from high- to low-risk populations along the routes of migration [74–79].

There is limited evidence in India on the movement/mobility-induced vulnerability of female sex workers [80–84]. The chance of economic improvement is a consistent motivation for movement among migrant communities across the globe, including India [76]. However, in the context of sex work, the reasons for mobility among female sex workers are varied. Recent studies on the mobility of female sex workers in southern India indicate that high interstate and district mobility is motivated by the need to earn more money in order to improve their economic condition and to repay debt [72]. The clandestine nature of sex work is another reason for female sex workers to change their sex work venues frequently. Change of place helps to avoid stigma and maintain secrecy about their work from family members [85].

Thus, female sex workers employ a number of strategies to continue their work despite the stigma associated with it. The example above illustrates how NGOs have organized different interventions including mobilizing and collectivization among others to prevent the transmission of HIV/STIs among sex workers and their clients. There is a clear need to design prevention interventions tailored to the needs of different female sex workers in different settings. The changing dynamics of client solicitation through mobile phones present new challenges for the design of appropriate interventions for mobilizing female sex workers and preventing the transmission of HIV/STIs.

References

1. Ditmore. Joint United Nations Programme on HIV/AIDS. UNAIDS; 2008.
2. Lafort Y, Geelhoed D, Cuma L, Lazaro CDM, Delva W, Luchters S, Temmerman M. Reproductive health services for populations at high risk of HIV: performance of a night clinic in Tete province, Mozambique. BMC Health Services Research; 2010.
3. Hawken MP, Melis RDJ, Ngombo DT, Mandaliya K, Ng'ang'a LW, Price J, Dallabetta G, Temmerman M. Part time female sex workers in a sub-urban community in Kenya: a vulnerable hidden population. Sex Transm Infect. 2002;78(4):271–73.
4. Buzdugan R, Copas A, Moses S, Blanchard J, Isac S, Ramesh BM, Washington R, Halli SS, Cowan FM. Devising a female sex work typology using data from Karnataka India. Int J Epidemiol. 2010;39(2):439–48.
5. Saggurti N, Verma RK, Halli SS, Swain SN, Singh R, Modugu HR, Ramarao S, Mahapatra B, Jain AK. Motivations for entry into sex work and HIV risk among mobile female sex workers in India. J Biosoc Sci. 2011;43(5):535–54.
6. Choi SYP. Heterogeneous and vulnerable: The health risks facing transnational female sex workers. Soc Health Illness. 2011;33(1):33–49.
7. World Health Organization. WHO consolidated guideline on self-care interventions for health: sexual and reproductive health and rights. Geneva: World Health Organization; 2019.
8. World Health Organization. Towards universal access: scaling up priority HIV/AIDS interventions in the health sector. Geneva: World Health Organization; 2009.
9. Prinja S, Bahuguna P, Rudra S, Gupta I, Kaur M, Mehendale SM, Chatterjee S, Panda S, Kumar R. Cost effectiveness of targeted HIV prevention interventions for female sex workers in India. Sex Transm Infect. 2011;87(4):354–61.
10. Pisani E. The wisdom of whores: Bureaucrats, brothels, and the business of AIDS. 2008.
11. Shannon K, Csete J. Violence, condom negotiation, and HIV/STI risk among sex workers. JAMA. 2010;304(5):573–4.
12. Wilson D. Access to HIV prevention, treatment, care and support for sex workers: report on the state of the art. PLoS Med. 2015.
13. Pettifor A, MacPhail C, Corneli A, Sibeko J, Kamanga G, Rosenberg N, Miller WC, Hoffman I, Rees H, Cohen MS. NIAID Center for HIV/AIDS vaccine immunology. Continuedhigh risk sexual behavior following diagnosis with acute HIV infection in South Africa and Malawi: implications for prevention. AIDS Behavior. 2011;15(6):1243–50.
14. Chakrapani V, Newman PA, Shunmugam M, Kurian AK, Dubrow R. Barriers to free antiretroviral treatment access for female sex workers in Chennai, India. AIDS Patient Care STDS. 2009;23(11):973–80.

15. Piot P. Setting new standards for targeted HIV prevention: the Avahan initiative in India. Sex Transm Infect. 2010;86(1):1–2.
16. Pillai S, Seshu M, Shivdas M. Embracing the rights of people in prostitution and sex workers, to address HIV and AIDS effectively. Gender Develop. 2008;16(2):313–26.
17. Gooptu N, Bandyopadhyay N. Rights to stop the wrong: Cultural change and collective mobilization—the case of Kolkata sex workers. Oxford Develop Study. 2007;35(3):251–72.
18. Reynaga E. Sex workers are part of the solution. Plenary presentation. UNESCO at the XVII International AIDS Conference, Mexico City. UNESDOC Digital Library. 2008.
19. National AIDS Control Organization. Annual Report 2015–2016. New Delhi: National AIDS Control Organization, Ministry of Health and Family Welfare, Government of India. 2016.
20. Blanchard JF, O'Neil J, Ramesh BM, Bhattacharjee P, Orchard T, Moses S. Understanding the social and cultural contexts of female sex workers in Karnataka, India: implications for prevention of HIV infection. J Infect Dis. 2005;191(1):139–46.
21. Shankar J. *Devadasi* cult: a sociological analysis. New Delhi: Ashish Publishing House; 1990.
22. Baral S, Beyrer C, Muessig K, Poteat T, Wirtz AL, Decker MR, Sherman SG, Kerrigan D. Burden of HIV among female sex workers in low-income and middle-income countries: a systematic review and meta-analysis. Lancet Infect Dis. 2012;12(7):538–49.
23. Shahmanesh M, Patel V, Mabey D, Cowan F. Effectiveness of interventions for the prevention of HIV and other sexually transmitted infections in female sex workers in resource poor setting: a systematic review. Tropical Med Int Health. 2008;13:659–79.
24. Silverman JG, Decker MR, Gupta J, Maheshwari A, Willis BM, Raj A. HIV prevalence and predictors of infection in sex-trafficked Nepalese girls and women. JAMA. 2007;298:536–42.
25. Wirtz A, Pretorius C, Sherman S, Baral S, Decker M, Sweat M, Kerrigan D. Modeling the impacts of a comprehensive community empowerment-based, HIV prevention intervention for female sex workers in generalized and concentrated epidemics: Infections averted among sex workers and adults. J Int AIDS Soc. 2012;15:107.
26. Swendeman D, Fehrenbacher AE, Ali S, George S, Mindry D, Collins M, Ghose T, Dey B. Whatever I have, I have made by coming into this profession: The intersection of resources, agency, and achievements in pathways to sex work in Kolkata, India. Archieves Sex Behav. 2015;44(4):1011–23.
27. Decker MR, Pearson E, Illangasekare SL, Clark E, Sherman SG. Violence against women in sex work and HIV risk implications differ qualitatively by perpetrator. BMC Public Health. 2013;23(13):876.
28. Deering KN, Amin A, Shoveller J, Nesbitt A, Garcia-Moreno C, Duff P, Argento E, Shannon K. A systematic review of the correlates of violence against sex workers. Am J Public Health. 2014;104(5):42–54.
29. Pando MA, Coloccini RS, Reynaga E, Rodriguez Fermepin M, Gallo Vaulet L, Kochel TJ, Montano SM, Avila MM. Violence as a barrier for HIV prevention among female sex workers in Argentina. PLoS ONE. 2013;8(1).
30. Beattie TS, Bhattacharjee P, Ramesh BM, Gurnani V, Anthony J, Isac S, Mohan HL, Ramakrishnan A, Wheeler T, Bradley J, Blanchard JF, Moses S. Violence against female sex workers in Karnataka state, South India: impact on health, and reductions in violence following an intervention program. BMC Public Health. 2010;10:476.
31. Wilson KS, Deya R, Masese L, Simoni JM, Stoep AV, Shafi J, Jaoko W, Hughes JP, McClelland RS. Prevalence and correlates of intimate partner violence in HIV-positive women engaged in transactional sex in Mombasa, Kenya. Int J STD AIDS. 2016;27(13):1194–203.
32. Ulibarri MD, Strathdee SA, Lozada R, Magis-Rodriguez C, Amaro H, O'Campo P & Patterson TL. Prevalence and correlates of client-perpetrated abuse among female sex workers in two Mexico-U.S. border cities. Violence Against Women. 2014;20(4):427–45.
33. Campbell J, Jones AS, Dienemann J, Kub J, Schollenberger J, O'Campo P, Gielen AC, Wynne C. Intimate partner violence and physical health consequences. Archieves Intern Med. 2002;162(10):1157–63.

34. Coker AL. Does physical intimate partner violence affect sexual health? A systematic review. Trauma Violence Abuse. 2007;8(2):149–77.
35. Campbell JC, Lucea MB, Stockman JK, Draughon JE. Forced sex and HIV risk in violent relationships. Am J Reprod Immunol New York. 2013;69:41–4.
36. Campbell JC. Health consequences of intimate partner violence. Lancet. 2002;359 (9314):1331–6.
37. Kouyoumdjian FG, Findlay N, Schwandt M, Calzavara LM. A systematic review of the relationships between intimate partner violence and HIV/AIDS. PLoS ONE. 2013;8 (11):81044.
38. Maman S, Campbell J, Sweat MD, Gielen AC. The intersections of HIV and violence: Directions for future research and interventions. Soc Sci Med. 2000;50(4):459–78.
39. Jewkes R. Intimate partner violence: causes and prevention. Lancet. 2002;359(9315):1423–9.
40. Dunkle KL, Jewkes RK, Brown HC, Gray GE, McIntryre JA, Harlow SD. Gender-based violence, relationship power, and risk of HIV infection in women attending antenatal clinics in South Africa. Lancet. 2004;363(9419):1415–21.
41. Rekart ML. Sex-work harm reduction. Lancet. 2005;366:2123–34.
42. Shannon K, Strathdee SA, Goldenberg SM, Duff P, Mwangi P, Rusakova M, Paul SR, Lau J, Deering K, Pickles MR, Boily MC. Global epidemiology of HIV among female sex workers: influence of structural determinants. Lancet. 2015;385(9962):55–71.
43. Basu I, Jana S, Rotheram-Borus MJ, Swendeman D, Lee SJ, Newman P, Weiss R. HIV prevention among sex workers in India. Jaids-J Acquir Immune Defic Syndr. 2004;36(3): 845–52.
44. Swendeman D, Basu I, Das S, Jana S, Rotheram-Borus MJ. Empowering sex workers in India to reduce vulnerability to HIV and sexually transmitted diseases. Soc Sci Med. 2009;69 (8):1157–66.
45. Fehrenbacher AE, Chowdhury D, Ghose T, Swendeman D. Consistent condom use by female sex workers in Kolkata, India: testing theories of economic insecurity, behavior change, life course vulnerability and empowerment. AIDS Behav. 2016;20(10):2332–45.
46. Ghose T, Swendeman D, George S, Chowdhury D. Mobilizing collective identity to reduce HIV risk among sex workers in Sonagachi, India: the boundaries, consciousness, negotiation framework. Soc Sci Med. 2008;67(2):311–20.
47. Kerrigan D, Ellen JA, Moreno L, Rosario S, Katz J, Celentano DD, Sweat M. Environmental-structural factors significantly associated with consistent condom use among female sex workers in the Dominican Republic. AIDS. 2003;17(3):415–23.
48. Gertler P, Shah M & Bertozzi SM. Risky business: the market for unprotected commercial sex. J Polit Econ. 2005;113(31).
49. Fehrenbacher AE, Chowdhury D, Jana S, Ray P, Dey B, Ghose T, Swendeman D. Consistent condom use by married and cohabiting female sex workers in India: investigating relational norms with commercial versus intimate partners. AIDS Behav. 2018;22(12):4034–47.
50. Mukandavire Z, Mitchell KM, Vickerman P. Comparing the impact of increasing condom use or HIV pre-exposure prophylaxis (PrEP) use among female sex workers. Epidemics. 2016;14:62–70.
51. Stoner BP, Whittington WLH, Aral SO, Hughes JP, Handsfield HH, Holmes KK. Avoiding risky sex partners: perception of partners' risks v. partners' self-reported risks. Sex Transm Infect. 2003;79(3):197–201.
52. Mahapatra B, Lowndes CM, Mohanty SK, Gurav K, Ramesh BM, Moses S, Washington R, Alary M. Factors associated with risky sexual practices among female sex workers in Karnataka, India. Plos One. 2013;8(4).
53. Wang C, Hawes SE, Gaye A, Sow PS, Ndoye I, Manhart LE, Wald A, Critchlow CW, Kiviat NB. HIV prevalence, previous HIV testing, and condom use with clients and regular partners among Senegalese commercial sex workers. Sex Transm Infect. 2007;83(7):534–40.
54. Elmes J, Nhongo K, Ward H, Hallett T, Nyamukapa C, White PJ, Gregson S. The price of sex: condom use and the determinants of the price of sex among female sex workers in Eastern Zimbabwe. J Infect Dis. 2014;1(210):569–78.

References

55. Kar SB, Pascual CA, Chickering KL. Empowerment of women for health promotion: a meta-analysis. Soc Sci Med. 1999;49:1431–60.
56. Jana S, Bandyopadhyay N, Mukherjee S, Dutta N, Basu I, Saha A. STD/HIV intervention with sex workers in West Bengal India. AIDS. 1998;12:101–8.
57. Swendeman DT, Jana S. The Sonagachi/Durbar programme: a prototype of a community-led structural intervention for HIV prevention. In: Parker R, editor. Structural interventions in public health. London: Routledge; 2013.
58. Parikh SA. The political economy of marriage and HIV: the ABC approach, "safe" infidelity, and managing moral risk in Uganda. Am J Public Health. 2007;97(7):1198–208.
59. Moret W. Economic strengthening for female sex workers: a review of the literature. ASPIRES, FHI 360, USA; 2014.
60. UNAIDS. Combination HIV prevention: tailoring and coordinating biomedical, behavioral and structural strategies to reduce new HIV infections. UNAIDS Discussion Paper, UNAIDS, Geneva; 2010.
61. UNAIDS. UNAIDS guidance note on HIV and sex work. UNAIDS, Geneva, Switzerland; 2012.
62. Bandura A. Self-efficacy: toward a unifying theory of behavioral change. Psychol Rev. 1977;84(2):191–215.
63. Galavotti C, Wheeler T, Kuhlmann AS, Saggurti N, Narayanan P, Kiran U, Dallabetta G. Navigating the swampy lowland: a framework for evaluating the effect of community mobilization in female sex workers in Avahan, the India AIDS initiative. J Epidemiol Commun Health. 2012;66(2):9–15.
64. Wheeler T, Kiran U, Dallabetta G, Jayaram M, Chandrasekaran P, Tangri A, Menon H, Kumta S, Sgaier S, Ramakrishnan A, Moore J, Wadhwani A, Alexander A. Learning about scale, measurement and community mobilisation: reflections on the implementation of the Avahan HIV/AIDS initiative in India. J Epidemiol Commun Health. 2012;66(2):16–25.
65. Blanchard AK, Mohan HL, Shahmanesh M, Prakash R, Isac S, Ramesh BM, Bhattacharjee P, Gurnani V, Moses S, Blanchard JF. Community mobilization, empowerment and HIV prevention among female sex workers in south India. BMC Public Health. 2013;16(13):234.
66. Boerma JT, Weir SS. Integrating demographic and epidemiological approaches to research on HIV/AIDS: the proximate-determinants framework. Int J Infect Dis. 2005;191(1):61–7.
67. Lagarde E, Schim van der Loeff M, Enel C, Holmgren B, Dray-Spira R, Pison G. Piau JP, Delaunay V, M'Boup S, Ndoye I, Coeuret-Pellicer M, Whittle H, Aaby P, MECORA Group. Mobility and the spread of human immunodeficiency virus into rural areas of West Africa. Int J Epidemiol. 2003;32(5):744–52.
68. Zaba B, Slaymaker E, Urassa M, Boerma JT. The role of behavioral data in HIV surveillance. AIDS. 2005;19(2):39–52.
69. Coffee M, Lurie MN, Garnett GP. Modelling the impact of migration on the HIV epidemic in South Africa. AIDS. 2007;21(3):343–50.
70. Rees D, Murray J, Nelson G, Sonnenberg P. Oscillating migration and the epidemics of silicosis, tuberculosis, and HIV infection in South African gold miners. Am J Ind Med. 2010;53(4):398–404.
71. International Organization for Migration. A behavioral study of female sex workers along Ghana's Tema-Paga Transport Corridor. IOM, Ghana; 2012.
72. Reed E, Gupta J, Biradavolu M, Blankenship KM. Migration/mobility and risk factors for HIV among female sex workers in Andhra Pradesh, India: implications for HIV prevention. Int J STD AIDS. 2012;23(4):7–13.
73. Guest P. Population mobility in Asia and implications for HIV/AIDS. Bangkok: UNDP South East Asia HIV and Development Project; 2000.
74. Thappa DM, Manjunath JV, Kartikeyan K. Truck drivers at increased risk of HIV infection amongst STD clinic attendees. Ind J Dermatol Venereol Leprol. 2002;68(5):312.
75. Singh S, Gupta K, Lahiri S, Schensul J. Dynamics of social networking, drug abuse and risk behaviour to STD and HIV/AIDS in India: a case study of adult male migrants in Surat, India.

Bio-statistical Aspects of Health and Population. New Delhi: Hindustan Publishing Corporation; 2006. p. 95–105.
76. Halli SS, Buzdugan R, Moses S, Blanchard J, Jain A, Verma R, Saggurti N. High-risk sex among mobile female sex workers in the context of jatras (religious festivals) in Karnataka, India. Int J STD AIDS. 2010;21(11):746–51.
77. Saggurti N, Schensul SL, Verma RK. Migration, mobility and sexual risk behavior in Mumbai, India: mobile men with non-residential wife show increased risk. AIDS Behav. 2009;13(5):921–7.
78. Saggurti N, Verma RK, Halli SS, Swain SN, Singh R, Modugu HR, Jain AK. Motivations for entry into sex work and HIV risk among mobile female sex workers in India. J Biosoc Sci. 2011;43(5):535–54.
79. Suryawanshi D, Sharma V, Saggurti N, Bharat S. Factors associated with the likelihood of further movement among mobile female sex workers in India: a multi-nominal logit approach. J Biosoc Sci. 2016;48(4):539–56.
80. Population Council. Patterns of migration/mobility and HIV risk among female sex workers: Andhra Pradesh. Population Council, New Delhi; 2008.
81. KHPT (Karnataka Health Promotion Trust) & Population Council. Patterns of migration/mobility and HIV risk among female sex workers: Karnataka. Karnataka Health Promotion Trust, Bangalore; 2008.
82. Verma RK, Saggurti N, Singh AK, Swain SN. Alcohol and sexual risk behavior among migrant female sex workers and male workers in districts with high in-migration from four high HIV prevalence states in India. AIDS Behav. 2010;14(1):31–9.
83. Ramesh S, Ganju D, Mahapatra B, Mishra R, Saggurti N. Relationship between mobility, violence and HIV/STI among female sex workers in Andhra Pradesh, India. BMC Public Health. 2012;12(1):1–8.
84. Saggurti N, Jain AK, Sebastian MP, Singh R, Modugu HR, Halli SS, Verma RK. Indicators of mobility, socio-economic vulnerabilities and HIV risk behaviours among mobile female sex workers in India. AIDS Behav. 2012;16(4):952–9.
85. Venkataramana C, Sarda P. Extent and speed of spread of HIV infection in India through the commercial sex networks: a perspective. Tropical Med Int Health. 2001;6(12):1040–61.

Open Access This chapter is licensed under the terms of the Creative Commons Attribution 4.0 International License (http://creativecommons.org/licenses/by/4.0/), which permits use, sharing, adaptation, distribution and reproduction in any medium or format, as long as you give appropriate credit to the original author(s) and the source, provide a link to the Creative Commons license and indicate if changes were made.

The images or other third party material in this chapter are included in the chapter's Creative Commons license, unless indicated otherwise in a credit line to the material. If material is not included in the chapter's Creative Commons license and your intended use is not permitted by statutory regulation or exceeds the permitted use, you will need to obtain permission directly from the copyright holder.

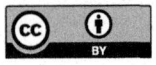

Chapter 5
Sexual Behaviors of Long-Distance Truck Drivers

5.1 Backdrop

Truck drivers are a group of recognized marginalized people who are sexually active during their long driving hours. Their exhausting working environment causing lethargy and mental fatigue stirs them to have sex [1]. Long-distance truck drivers transport goods over hundreds and even thousands of miles. They may drive flatbed rigs, which are used for carrying steel, or tankers and tractor trailers. They usually drive at night when traffic is light [2]. Truck drivers and interstate migrants are important bridge populations for the transmission of HIV infection [3].

Since truckers travel long distances, they are away from home for extended periods of time and so they interact with sex workers along their travel routes [4, 5]. Truckers are vulnerable to the human immunodeficiency virus (HIV) and other sexually transmitted infections (STIs) [6]. Truckers in India and in many other countries are known to suffer from and transmit HIV/STIs [7]. To prevent infection transmission, it is important to understand the complexity of their sexual behaviors by developing a framework for the prevention of HIV/STIs [8, 9].

Truck drivers are at risk of several health problems including diabetes and cardiovascular diseases [10]. Truckers who get infected with HIV/STIs while traveling carry back these infections to their wives [11, 12]. They acquire these infections on their travels but specially at places where their trucks are loaded and unloaded and where their documentation is inspected [7].

Mobility is a major factor for the spread of sexually transmitted infections like HIV across different geographical locations [1]. Prevalence of diseases like HIV is more common in people living in rural settings, especially in areas which are populated along the roads, because of low income, lack of education, and awareness about barrier contraception and use of condoms [13]. Studies suggest that unmarried truck drivers, those who drink alcohol, those who stay away from home for more than 15 days, and middle-income drivers are significantly more likely to visit female sex workers than married drivers [14].

5.2 Research on Long-Distance Truck Drivers

Research was undertaken to study the values, preferences, and practices with regard to self-care for sexual and reproductive health and rights (SRHR) and HIV prevention and treatment in long-distance truck drivers. The objectives were to obtain an understanding of their views about self-care practices; how they obtained information on self-care interventions; what were their motivations to use them; what barriers they faced while using them; and what they did if self-care practices failed.

Research was undertaken in Delhi and Tamil Nadu. A qualitative study design was employed. In-depth interviews (IDIs), focus group discussions (FGDs), key informant interviews (KIIs), and a workshop were conducted with long-distance truck drivers. Qualitative research methods allowed greater spontaneity and interaction with participants. They provided an opportunity to the participants to respond elaborately and in greater detail. The interviews were conducted using interview guides. The interviews were approximately 90–120 minutes in length. The interviews were recorded, and the recordings were transcribed and checked for accuracy. Four IDIs, two KIIs, and two FGDs (8–10 participants) were conducted in Delhi. One workshop was conducted in Tamil Nadu with 24 long-distance truck drivers to understand their general health problems, sexual health and HIV issues, and how they accessed information on SRH products and services on social media and other platforms.

For the key informant interviews, participants were selected on the basis of their experience. They were peer educators working with NGOs. For in-depth interviews, outreach workers with 4–5 years of experience were selected. Focus group discussions included peer educators, outreach workers, and other young long-distance truck drivers. During the workshop, participants were asked to depict their sexual practices in art form for which they were provided with colors and canvas.

Triangulation of data generated by KIIs, IDIs, FGDs, and the workshop made it possible to obtain reliable information on complex issues. Ethical approval for undertaking the study was granted by the Ethical Review Board of the Humsafar Trust. Before initiating the study, participants were given consent forms which described the study. Consent of all participants was taken in writing and orally. Confidentiality of all participants was assured.

5.2.1 Research Findings

The findings include a discussion of the lifestyle and behaviors of long-distance truck drivers; self-care interventions for SRHR; information sources for SRHR; risks and barriers faced by the community; and motivations for self-care.

5.2.2 Lifestyle of Long-Distance Truck Drivers

The lives of truck drivers were not easy. A lot of hard work, patience, and perseverance was needed. They had difficult long hours on the road (Fig. 5.1).

> Our profession is unique; we are responsible for other peoples' lives.

On their long journeys, they got little or no sleep. They were stressed and worn down with the difficult conditions on the road that they faced with their jobs.

> We have no life, people do not respect us. Our life is like a long lonely haul.

Truck drivers had less stability in life as they traveled for several days continuously to transport their cargo on time, without any rest and sleep.

> We are not here willingly; difficult conditions at home force us to become truckers.

They preferred to have processed food and sugary beverages while traveling which caused adverse effects. At times, they did not even get water to clean themselves.

> We do not have access to proper food, rest and sanitation.

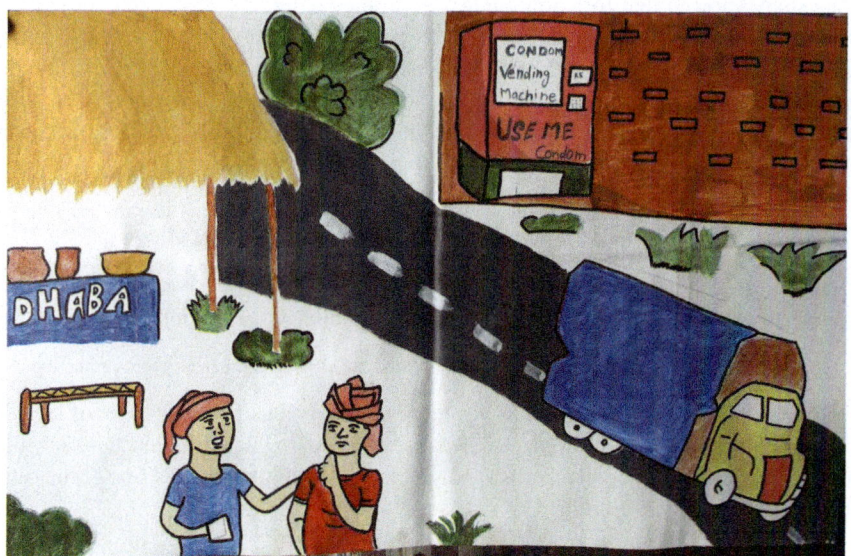

Fig. 5.1 Truck drivers stop at a Dhaba painting by Karan

5.2.3 Sexual Behaviors of Long-Distance Truck Drivers

Truck drivers, a mobile population, traveled long distances and were away from home for months. The intersection of truck drivers with female sex workers was very common. They often had sexual encounters with female sex workers without any protection, and so they were at high risk of HIV.

> We prefer to have sex with female sex workers and transgender on our route as they carry condoms with them.

They had great faith in their family doctors whom they consulted with some regularity. They followed their family doctor's advice with regard to adopting/using health products and services. When on the road long-distance truck routes, they carried previously issued prescriptions prepared by their family doctors and reused them to buy medicines from pharmacies. They typically followed their family doctor's advice in whom they had great faith.

> Whenever we go home, we visit our family doctor. We do not like to visit any other doctor en route. If we have some problem, we take the medicines we have or use the prescriptions given by our family doctor.

5.2.4 Self-care Interventions for Sexual and Reproductive Health

The study showed that for common health problems, like headache and body ache, truck drivers often used topical pain relief, painkiller tablets, and sprays. For fever, diarrheal diseases, abdominal pain, and other such problems, truck drivers bought medicines from a pharmacy or from a private practitioner. Their ability to visit practitioners was dependent on the availability of time and access. They found it difficult to access practitioners when driving on long-distance routes.

> We have to unload the material in the given time, so we prefer not to stop the truck in between even if we are not feeling well.

They used condoms when they had sex with female sex workers and transgender. Female sex workers and transgender usually brought condoms with them.

> Sex workers usually carry condoms. They do not allow us to be intimate without protection.

The use of gels and creams was very rare among truck drivers because of lack of knowledge. The study showed that because of their regular drinking habits while driving, truckers frequently had sexual encounters without protection. Some also had sex with their helpers.

> Sometimes we forcefully have sex with our helpers when drunk.

5.2.5 Information Sources

Truck drivers revealed that it was really very important for them to have knowledge about HIV prevention and sexual and reproductive health. They got their information through their interpersonal contact with their peers as well as peer educators and outreach workers. They also got information related to condom use for safe sex from them (Fig. 5.2).

> Our fellow drivers are an important source of health information. We gather information from peers especially about common health problems such as painful micturition, ulcers and blisters, and muscular pain and take medication based on their advice.

The study showed that they trusted health-related information or products and services that they received via social media, e.g., Facebook and WhatsApp. All the truck drivers had smartphones. They did not watch television regularly. But when they did, they did not trust health product or service-related advertisements seen on television.

> Because of lack of time, we do not access social media or television for information related to sexual and reproductive health.

NGOs provided condom demonstrations and information on hygienic practices but because they traveled, not every trucker received this information. It was also

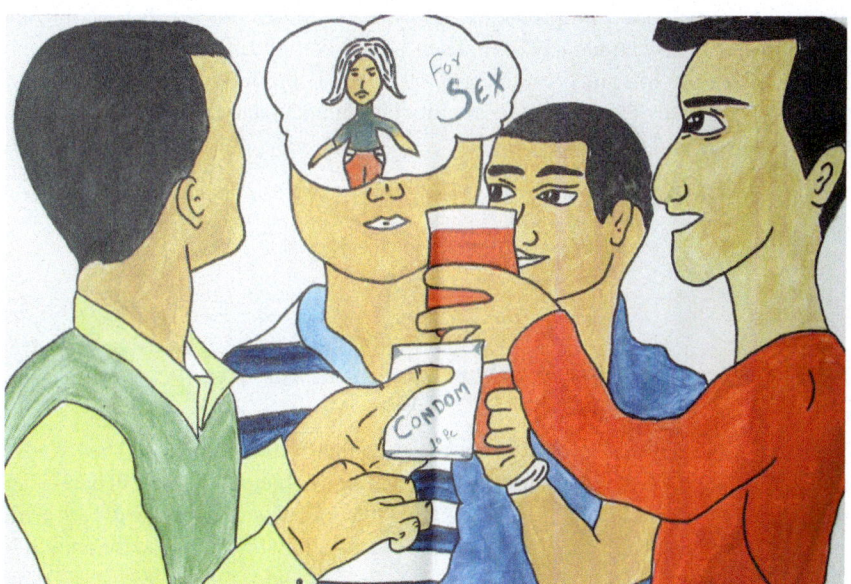

Fig. 5.2 Truck drivers sharing information painting by Karan

found that truckers visited private doctors for health-related problems and had to spend a lot for these consultations.

> We do not have time to visit public facilities. We have to visit private physicians, and we end up spending a huge amount.

5.2.6 Issues Related to Cost and Affordability

Being a truck driver was a very grueling job. Truck drivers had unattractive careers and poor pay. They led unhealthy lifestyles. Sometimes, they had no work for many days, and they suffered from bankruptcy.

> We are disadvantaged because of lack of knowledge; doctors charge us more for providing medicine. They charge Rs. 500 for a medicine that costs Rs. 10.

5.2.7 Risks and Barriers Faced by the Community

The study showed that the truckers had sex most frequently with female sex workers and transgender. They had poor knowledge about sexual and reproductive health. They faced difficulties because of their long journeys and not being at home. There was poor availability of public toilets en route, and so they suffered from illness and sexual health problems. They had limited knowledge about self/user-initiated interventions (S/UIIs). They feared complications due to inappropriate use of testing kits, medication, and other S/UII products and services. Given their limited literacy levels, they faced difficulty in understanding which products or services to use and how to use them.

> It is very difficult to access proper medical care as we travel long distance highway routes. Language changes as we cross state borders. Therefore, we always carry old prescriptions to get medication from pharmacies when en route our travel.

5.2.8 Mental Health Problems and Violence

The study revealed that most truckers faced mental health problems. They were at risk for a range of occupational health conditions, including mental health and psychiatric disorders due to high occupational stress, low access and use of health care, and limited social support. They were exposed to violence and were abused by the owners, police, and others.

> Many times police charge a fine for no reason, and we have to pay from our pocket.

They suffered physical illness, mental illness, and addictions of habit-forming substances, specially tobacco. Because of their long journeys, they rarely visited their homes, and so faced isolation and sometimes depression. At times, they went for days without work which also caused depression. Some became alcoholics.

> We face stress on a daily basis due to long working hours and end up with the habits of regular smoking and alcohol.

5.2.9 Motivations for Self-care

The study showed that truckers were less motivated and unaware about their physical and mental health and well-being. They had limited knowledge about sexual and reproductive health. They forced female sex workers to have sex without protection when they were drunk. NGOs organized workshops to improve the self-care practices of truckers but as they had mobile jobs, they were not always available to attend these workshops and so were left with limited information. They were motivated to access self-testing kits (e.g., STI self-testing kits). Since they were illiterate, they were not able to follow directions for use provided with these kits. NGOs motivated them to access STI and HIV self-testing and treatment, so that they could use these products at their discretion.

5.2.10 A Personal Narrative by a Member of the Trucking Community

Documented By: Dr. Rashmi Pachauri Rajan

I see myself as an agent of change who embraced the tenets of self-care early in life. I began my career with a high school diploma and had practically no knowledge of sexual and reproductive health care. I live in Sanjay Gandhi Transport Nagar, also known as SGTN, the largest trucking halt point in Asia, covering 77 acres, where at any given point, there are at least 73,000 trucks. It is a halt point—a pickup, drop-off, and loading point for truck drivers. This community also includes helpers, mechanics, insurance and booking agents, and labor contractors. It was one of the first demonstration sites for interventions at the height of the HIV movement in India in the early 2000s. This movement created, over time, a number of community leaders among the truck driver community, of whom I am one.

I began working as a "helper" (a young assistant of truck drivers, also referred to as a "cleaner"). My job included cleaning the vehicle, helping with its maintenance, watching over the truck and its cargo, and doing other odd jobs. But since I was only called three to four times a month to undertake journeys from Delhi to Kanpur (a distance of 496 km), I also continued to run my own tea stall in the same area.

As part of this community, I saw closely the lifestyle of the drivers and helpers—their long-distance relationships with their families, their frequent dependence on alcohol and drugs, their unsafe sexual activity on the road, their having to deal frequently with police and abuse. I noted the tremendous risks they took because of the brutality of their lifestyle, their illiteracy, ignorance, and disregard for safety.

While working in SGTN, after persistence and perseverance, I got an additional job as a peer educator with a nonprofit organization based in the same area. There, I underwent intense training on interpersonal and peer-to-peer communication and counseling for HIV prevention. I learned about the use and importance of condoms, emergency contraceptives, and abortion pills. This was a turning point in my life, as the information I gained enhanced my ability to practice self-care in all its various forms. I am now a proud Project Officer at an education, training, and research institution and work nationally. In this leadership position, I am able to spread knowledge on self-care to peers, family, friends, and the larger community.

I am in a long-term relationship, which is uncommon within the community. I am particular about using condoms. I provide my partner with emergency contraception. I have self-tested for HIV and advise my partner to do the same. I advise friends and peers who come to me for information on unwanted pregnancy, sexually transmitted infections, and HIV prevention and testing. I feel I am an exception within the community which is otherwise, still negligent with respect to health. It is fatalistic and, therefore, less likely and even resistant to adopting self-care strategies, especially in the sphere of sexual and reproductive health.

However, I do have some concerns about self-care products because the instruction leaflets for these products are often in English and cannot be understood by those not proficient in the language. These instructions must be regionally translated. Today, even the illiterate and the poor own smartphones and are tech-savvy enough to be able to Google or obtain information from the Internet (e.g., YouTube). It would therefore be useful if product instructions included information to source appropriate videos on YouTube.

Over the last decade, I have come a long way. I am now a community leader and am proud that my learnings and knowledge have made me aware of the crucial importance of self-care I can assist my community in the planning, implementation, and monitoring of key programs—a major step forward to achieving the goal of universal health coverage.

> Self-care has been practiced over the years. It is now formally recognized by the World Health Organization (WHO) that when self-care interventions are accessible and affordable, they "have the potential to increase choice, as well as opportunities for individuals to make informed decisions regarding their health and health care. Approaches that facilitate user autonomy and peer support have the potential to advance health through strategies that promote participation of individuals in their own health care." One of WHO's "triple billion" goals is to achieve Universal Health Coverage, which necessitates that health needs of vulnerable populations be met.

5.2.11 A Long-Distance Truck Driver's Personal Narrative on Self-care

Documented By: Philo Magdalene A.

Professional truck drivers in India live through demanding labor conditions that tend to compromise their basic health behaviors, making them a community with heightened vulnerabilities in terms of physical and mental health. Twenty-eight-year-old Sahabudin from Haryana helps bring this perspective as he recounts his journey as a truck driver.

When asked about how he feels about his life after becoming a truck driver, he sighs, *"To be honest, there is no life since the day I decided to do this job. At home, nobody thinks about becoming a truck driver, but only after becoming one does one realize that he should never have opted for this job."* Sahabudin dropped out of school after 5th class, and seeing that his father struggled to provide for his family *from* being just a laborer, he decided to become more productive. He started learning to drive trucks in his late teenage years and became a professional truck driver by the time he turned twenty.

His discontent stems from many factors that essentially relate to his work. Driving round-the-clock for as long as five days always results in physical exhaustion causing back pain and headaches. On a normal day, he takes turns with his co-driver to break for rest and eat at the highway *dhabas* en route. These *dhabas* are heavily relied upon by many truck drivers as they have clean toilet facilities that are otherwise difficult to find within a 30–40 km radius. Sahabudin says that oftentimes they are forced to use the bushes due to lack of water facilities in the region they travel. Even though the number of toll plazas they cross during their journey is numerous, they are hardly of any help, as the toilets in toll plazas are either not cleaned or do not have water. These factors also prevent them from bathing regularly between destinations.

The roads decide access to food and clean toilets for the drivers who are constantly on the move, adding uncertainty to their basic health routines. In addition to this vulnerability, one can understand from Sahabudin that there are other difficulties that accompany his job. Police harassment of truck drivers has become a normalized behavior that every truck driver has to go through silently. *"On the Rajasthan-Jaipur road, there are so many RTOs (Regional Transport Officers) who check my truck, and even when it is not overloaded, they take money from me like 500 to 1000 rupees. If I do not give them the money, they beat me,"* says Sahabudin. Truck drivers also deal with the risk of thieves in regions like Madhya Pradesh where they avoid driving at night to ensure their safety.

It is important to note that this growing list of challenges is not all that paints the job of a truck driver. There are some positive aspects also, and Sahabudin speaks of how the drivers develop a good relationship with people they meet in the little *dhabas* on the road who act as their safety net whenever they require roadside assistance in times of any emergency. The employer is also considered as their support system as he ensures that the drivers return home immediately in case of any personal emergency. Furthermore, Sahabudin has not faced any financial difficulty so far when it comes to meeting his medical needs because, as he says, *"Our boss makes sure that nobody falls ill, and even if we fall ill, he helps us in getting treatment."*

He, along with other truck drivers, carries minimal belongings for the road. Medicines are bought from village doctors prior to the journey, as they avoid buying medicines when on the road. Sahabudin adds that they also refrain from visiting doctors outside their region because of the difficulty in communication due to the language barrier. The doctors back home are consulted, even remotely, when any need arises. When asked about purchasing medicines and storing them for the journey, Sahabudin responds, *"We don't buy medicines in bulk. If somebody falls ill and we know that we have the medicine for that ailment, we give it to him. But we don't store medicines for a very long time."*

Government hospitals in cities like Delhi provide the kind of care that is difficult for Sahabudin to find or afford in his hometown. He does not own a health card sanctioned by the government because he claims that his community does not believe in doing a postmortem when a person dies in an accident as it is against their religion. When asked if the same logic applies to the use of contraceptives, he says, *"First of all, our religion forbids us to go outside our marriage and have sex with other people's wives. And if you dare to go without a condom, and she has a child, it is a sinful act."*

HIV and AIDS are *terminologies* that are not new to them. It is, in fact, *"the most common talk amongst drivers"* according to Sahabudin. Yet, when probed about the extent of his awareness with regard to HIV/AIDS, he says, *"This information is enough for us to know that if we do it outside (marriage), we might end up having some problem."* Questions about his sexual health are similarly fielded as Sahabudin, who says that only an "unmarried" individual can/should talk about contraceptives and sexual life, pointing to the unmarried driver next to him.

Sahabudin's companion *discloses* that they do not have any obligation to carry condoms with them because the sex workers never fail to *bring* condoms. They are very particular in this regard, often refusing to engage with the customer in the absence of a contraceptive. He also notes that the sex workers, who are fully supported by the members of their families, live with them in colonies on the outskirts of Rajasthan and Madhya Pradesh, and it is common to see the truck drivers marry into these families.

Being distanced from home for prolonged periods of time and constant worrying about the welfare of their loved ones add to their mental stress and physical burnout. Light physical activities and mental diversions through phone calls are the only plausible ways available to them to deal with this overwhelming stress. Sahabudin understands the need to take care of his body, especially during times of illness, because, like every other truck driver, he has a responsibility towards his family. If he gets unwell, "the whole family will crumble." For Sahabudin, whose job vulnerabilities risk every aspect of his life, following the everyday basic health routine is a form of self-care that he believes he should rely on.

5.3 Discussion

The trucking population in India is estimated as 5–6 million truckers and helpers of which 2.5 million are long-distance truck drivers [15, 16]. Research shows that long-distance truck drivers have sex with female sex workers and also with unpaid partners [3, 17]. Consistent condom use is low (58–74%) with the former and with the latter (20%) [3, 18–20]. The prevalence of HIV (2–13%) and STIs (3–16%) is high among long-distance truck drivers [3, 19, 21, 22].

Risky sexual behavior and prevalence of HIV/STIs in truck drivers depend on several factors including age, education, marital status, duration away from home, and alcohol intake [3, 17–23]. Studies show that in India unmarried truck drivers are more likely than married truck drivers to have risky sexual behaviors. They also have early sexual debut—before reaching 18 years [17, 21–25]. Studies in other countries also show that earlier initiation of sexual intercourse is associated with higher risk-taking in truck drivers [26–29].

Research indicates that very few married truckers report consistent condom use with their wives. This could be due to greater level of intimacy and trust in such relationships, lower risk perception among married drivers, and also the perception of condoms as a means of family planning and not as a measure to prevent STIs and HIV. Inconsistent condom use among the married truck drivers put their wives at risk of getting infected with STIs and HIV. These findings provide empirical evidence to show that long-distance truck drivers are an important bridge population for the transmission of HIV and STIs from the high-risk group of commercial sex workers to the low-risk group of general women.

Research showed that there was a highly significant relationship between alcohol intake and female sex worker exposure. Those who consumed alcohol were 2.71 times more likely to visit a commercial sex worker than those who did not [30]. High alcohol consumption (87%) among truck drivers is reported by several researchers [24, 31, 32].

Due to the nature of their profession, long-distance truck drivers have to stay away from home for long periods of time. They traverse the length and breadth of the country. Being in the sexually active age group, their exposure to female sex workers is frequent. These factors make them an epidemiologically important risk group for the transmission of HIV infection. Thus, changing their sexual behavior is of paramount importance to protect these drivers and prevent the spread of HIV infection. A highly significant relationship was found between the number of days spent outside home and exposure to female sex workers. Truck drivers who stayed away for more than 20 days from their homes were 15 times more likely to have exposure to female sex workers [6].

The trucking industry in India is largely unorganized and almost entirely in the private domain, structured around a loose system comprising truck operators, intermediaries, and users. In the late 1990s, almost 77% of India's truck fleet was owned by operators with no more than five trucks, whereas only about 6% was owned by operators with more than 20 trucks [7]. The highest risk of HIV occurs in places where trucks are loaded and unloaded, or where truck drivers stop to have their documentation inspected (which can take a considerable length of time). Long-haul truck drivers and their commercial sex contacts (the women and men with whom they exchange money and/or drugs for sex) have been implicated in the spread of HIV and other sexually transmitted infections (STIs) along major transportation routes in developing countries [33]. Studies in India have found high HIV (2–13%) and high STI prevalence (3–16%) in long-distance truck drivers [21, 32, 34].

A number of studies in India show that long-distance truck drivers have sexual intercourse with female sex workers, but most of them do not use condoms or use them infrequently [35–37]. Only consistent and correct use of condoms offers effective prevention against STIs [21]. Condom education and promotions should therefore be integrated with other HIV prevention strategies to address a range of behaviors in truck drivers.

A study by Chaturvedi et al. in 2006 showed that truck drivers who were away from home for more than 20 days were 15 times more likely to have exposure to female sex workers [20]. This is probably due to the fact that they were away from their regular sex partners for long durations. Most of the truck drivers were exposed to female sex worker along the roadside *dhabas* (small restaurants) on the highway. There were multiple reasons for not using condoms while having sex with female sex workers. These were non-availability, uneasy feeling (decreased pleasure), or unnecessary, similar to the finding of studies done by Pandey et al. [34] and McCree et al. [38]. Programs targeted to STI prevention should not only encourage condom use, but also make sure of the availability of condoms by placing vending machines in the *dhabas* which are located along the highways.

Herget reported a prevalence of 13% of truckers and their wives ever engaging in anal intercourse which was relatively high, given the sociocultural and legal context of sexual behaviors in India, where anal sex is considered non-normative, heavily stigmatized, and criminal under Section 377 of Indian Penal Code 63 (repealed by the Delhi High Court in July 2009 for consensual anal sex between adults) [39, 40]. The sexual experience of married women in India is generally influenced by gender power relations, cultural expectations, marital sexual relationships, and perceptions of appropriate male and female behaviors [41]. It is possible that the women in the study were coerced into anal intercourse by their husbands. However, the association between marital relationship attitudes or sexual relationship control and reporting of anal intercourse by the wives was not significant.

Research shows that younger couples were more likely to engage in anal intercourse. This could be because younger couples are more exposed to social media and are more open to experimentation [42]. Another hypothesis is that they avoid vaginal intercourse to prevent pregnancy. Yet another explanation is that they prefer anal intercourse because they can enjoy sexual pleasure without using condoms not recognizing that anal sex increases the risk of HIV/STIs [43]. It is also possible that some of these men might have a homosexual orientation but are married due to social pressure [44]. Additionally, it is widely believed that HIV is transmitted by vaginal intercourse, so it is not necessary to use condoms for anal sex [45–47].

The Avahan intervention with long-distance truck drivers began in 2004. To enhance accessibility of clinical services to truckers *Khushi* (meaning "happiness" in Hindi/Urdu), clinics were established at 36 truck halt points. This intervention was redesigned in 2006 by halving the numbers of implementation sites from 36 to 17 focusing on the major truck halt points in nine Indian states. It was revamped to take advantage of the structure of the Indian trucking industry with middlemen where truckers spend time between shipments. Peer educators recruited for the project increased the emphasis on professional media including mid-media and mass media events improved signage and satellite clinical services at the halt points [23, 48].

The Avahan intervention was evaluated to assess whether highways had become "safer" in terms of risk of HIV transmission among truckers. Safer highways meant increase in exposure to HIV prevention interventions and consistent condom use with non-regular female sexual partners along with a reduction in sexually transmitted infections including HIV among truckers [49].

There was an overall improvement in safe sexual practices with the increasing program exposure among long-distance truck drivers in the country. The program was able to reach those truckers who took higher risks, and once exposed to the intensive program these high-risk truckers were more likely to follow safe sexual practices by using condoms every time in all commercial sex acts. Interventions targeted to female sex workers also contributed to bringing about safe sexual practices among truckers [50].

Long-distance truck drivers constitute an important bridge population for the transmission of STIs including HIV. Long, arduous journeys across the land keep them away from home for lengths of time. Alcohol drinking is another common feature of that lifestyle. These factors contribute to truck drivers having sex with female sex workers en route. Research shows that while most truck drivers have sexual encounters with female sex workers, the majority of these are without protection resulting in a high incidence of HIV and other STIs. Programs designed to provide HIV prevention interventions on the highway have proven to improve sexual practices among long-distance truck drivers, thereby reducing the prevalence of STIs and HIV. Self-care by consistent condom use by truckers led to decreased prevalence of infection and its spread.

References

1. Essuon AD, Simmons DS, Stephens TT, Richter D, Lindley LL, Braithwaite RL. Transient populations: Linking HIV, migrant workers, and South African male inmates. J Health Care Poor Underserved. 2009;20:40–52.
2. American Trucking Associations. Long-haul truck driver: definition and nature of work. American Trucking Associations, Encyclopedia. 2020.

3. Pandey A, Benara SK, Roy N, Sahu D, Thomas M, Joshi DK, Sengupta U, Paranjape RS, Bhalla A, Prakash A, IBBA Study Team. Risk behaviour, sexually transmitted infections and HIV among long-distance truck drivers: a cross-sectional survey along national highways in India. AIDS. 2008;22(5):81–90.
4. Chandrasekaran P, Dallabetta G, Loo V, Rao S, Gayle H, Alexander A. Containing HIV/AIDS in India: the unfinished agenda. Lancet Infect Dis. 2006;6:508–21.
5. O'Neil J, Orchard T, Swarankar RC, Blanchard JF, Gurav K, Dhandha MS. Dharma and disease: traditional sex work and HIV/AIDS in rural India. Soc Sci Med. 2004;59:851–60.
6. Chaturvedi S, Banerjee A, Khera A, Joshi R, Dhrubajyoti D. Sexual behaviour among long distance truck drivers. Ind J Commun Med. 2006;31.
7. Thakur A, Toppo M, Lodha R. A study on sexual risk behaviors of long-distance truck drivers in central India. Int J Res Med Sci. 2017;3(7):1769–74.
8. Aral SO. Sexual risk behaviour and infection: epidemiological considerations. Sex Transm Infect. 2004;80:8–12.
9. Hayes R, Kapiga S, Padian N, McCormack S, Wasserheit JN. HIV prevention research: taking stock and the way forward. AIDS. 2010;24:81–92.
10. Greenfield R, Busink E, Wong CP, Riboli-Sasco E, Greenfield G, Majeed A, Car J, Wark PA. Truck drivers' perceptions on wearable devices and health promotion: a qualitative study. BMC Public Health. 2016;16(1):677.
11. Singh YN, Malaviya AN. Long distance truck drivers in India: HIV infection and their possible role in disseminating HIV into rural areas. Int J STD AIDS. 1994;5:137–8.
12. Steinbrook R. HIV in India: a complex epidemic. N Engl J Med. 2007;356:1089–93.
13. Yaya I, Landoh DE, Saka B, Vignikin K, Aboubakari AS, N'dri KM, Gbetoglo KD, Edorh AM, Ahlegnan K, Yenkey H, Toudeka AS, Pitche P. Consistent condom use during casual sex among long-truck drivers in Togo. PloS ONE. 2016;11:0.
14. Singh RK, Joshi HS. Sexual behavior among truck drivers. Ind J Public Health. 2012;56(1):53–6.
15. National AIDS Control Organization (NACO), Ministry of Health & Family Welfare & Government of India. Targeted intervention for truckers: operational guidelines, NACP III. New Delhi, NACO; 2007.
16. National Institute of Medical Statistics (NIMS) & National AIDS Control Organization (NACO). Technical report, India HIV estimates-2006. New Delhi: Ministry of Health and Family Welfare; 2006.
17. Bryan AD, Fisher JD, Benziger TJ. Determinants of HIV risk among Indian truck drivers. Soc Sci Med. 2001;53:1413–26.
18. Kumar S, Garg SK, Bajpai SK. A study of knowledge, sexual behavior and practices regarding HIV/AIDS among long distance truck drivers. Ind J Public Health. 2009;53:243–5.
19. Dude A, Oruganti G, Kumar V, Mayer KH, Yeldandi V, Schneider JA. HIV infection, genital symptoms and sexual risk behavior among Indian truck drivers from a large transportation company in south India. J Glob Infect Dis. 2009;1:21–8.
20. Chaturvedi S, Singh Z, Banerjee A, Khera A, Joshi RK, Dhrubajyoti D. Sexual behaviour among long distance truck drivers. Ind J Commun Med. 2006;31:153–6.
21. Bal B, Ahmed SI, Mukherjee R, Chakraborty S, Niyogi SK, Talukder A, Chakraborty N, Sarkar K. HIV infection among transport workers operating through Siliguri-Guwahati national highway. India. J Int Assoc Phys AIDS Care. 2007;6:56–60.
22. Manjunath JV, Thappa DM, Jaisankar TJ. Sexually transmitted diseases and sexual lifestyles of long-distance truck drivers: a clinico-epidemiologic study in South India. Int J STD AIDS. 2002;13:612–7.
23. Bill & Melinda Gates Foundation (BMGF). Off the beaten track: Avahan's experience in the business of HIV prevention among India's long-distance truckers, New Delhi, India. The Bill & Melinda Gates Foundation; 2008.
24. Bansal RK. Truck drivers and risk of STDs including HIV. Ind J Commun Med. 1995;20:28–30.

References

25. Family Health International, Department for International Development. Summary report: Behavioral surveillance survey in healthy highway project, India. New Delhi: Family Health International, DFID; 2001.
26. Collumbien M, Das B, Bohider N. Male sexual debut in Orissa, India: context, partners and differentials. Asia Pac Popul J. 2001;16:211–24.
27. Coker AL, Richter DL, Valois RF, McKeown RE, Garrison CZ, Vincent ML. Correlates and consequences of early initiation of sexual intercourse. J School Health. 1994;64:372–7.
28. White R, Cleland J, Carael M. Links between premarital sexual behavior and extramarital intercourse: a multi-site analysis. AIDS. 2000;14:2323–31.
29. Pettifor A, O'Brien K, Macphail C, Miller WC, Rees H. Early coital debut and associated HIV risk factors among young women and men in South Africa. Int Perspect Sex Reprod Health. 2009;35:82–90.
30. Pandey A, Mishra RM, Sahu D, Benara SK, Biswas M, Sengupta U, Mainkar MK, Adhikary R. Heterosexual risk behaviour among long distance truck drivers in India: role of marital status. Ind J Med Res. 2012;136(7):44.
31. Rao KS, Pilli RD, Rao AS, Chalam PS. Sexual behavior among long distance truck drivers. BMJ Suppl. 1999;318:162–3.
32. Manjunath J, Thappa D, Jaishankar T. Sexually transmitted disease and sexual lifestyle of long-distance lorry drivers: a clinical-epidemiological study in South India. Int J STD AIDS. 2002;13:612–7.
33. Alam N, Rahman M, Gausia K, Yunus MD, Islam N, Chaudhury P, Monira S, Funkhouser E, Vermund SH, Killewo J. Sexually transmitted infections and risk factors among truck stand workers in Dhaka, Bangladesh. Sex Transm Dis. 2007;34:99–103.
34. Pandey A, Mishra RM, Sahu D, Benara SK, Biswas M, Sengupta U, Mainkar MK, Adhikary R. Heterosexual risk behavior among long distance truck drivers in India: role of marital status. Ind J Med Res. 2012;136(7):44.
35. Singh YNK. Singh R, Joshi GK, Rustagi & Malaviya AN. HIV infection among long-distance truck drivers in Delhi, India. J Acquir Immune Defic Syndr. 1993;6(3):323.
36. Ahmed SI. Truck drivers as a vulnerable group in North-East India. In: Aggarwal OP, Sharma AK, Indrayan. A HIV/AIDS research in India, NACO, Ministry of Health & Family Welfare, Govt. of India; 1997, p. 497.
37. Mishra R. STD and HIV/AIDS: A KAP study among truck operators. Health Millions. 1998;224(5):11–3.
38. McCree DH, Cosgrove S, Stratford D, Valway S, Keller N, Hernandez JV, Jenison SA. Sexual and drug use risk behaviors of long-haul truck drivers and their commercial sex contacts in New Mexico. Public Health Rep. 2010;125(1):52–60.
39. Herget G. India: UNAIDS claims law criminalizing homosexuality hinders HIV prevention. HIV AIDS Policy Law Rev. 2006;11:35–6.
40. 2009 Judgement on IPC Section 377. Gay and transgender rights in India. Naz Foundation; 2009.
41. George A. Differential perspectives of men and women in Mumbai, India on sexual relations and negotiations within marriage. Reprod Health Matters. 1998;6:87–96.
42. Verma RK, Mahendra VS. Construction of masculinity in India: a gender and sexual health perspective. J Fam Welf. 2004;50:71–8.
43. Tian LH, Peterman TA, Tao G, Brooks LC, Metcalf C, Malotte CK, Paul SM, Douglas JM, RESPECT-2 Study Group. Heterosexual anal sex activity in the year after an STD clinic visit. Sex Transm Dis. 2008;35:905–9.
44. Solomon SS, Mehta SH, Latimore A, Srikrishnan AK, Celentano DD. The impact of HIV and high-risk behaviors on the wives of married men who have sex with men and injection drug users: Implications for HIV prevention. J Int AIDS Soc. 2010;13:7.
45. Bhattacharya G. Sociocultural and behavioral contexts of condom use in heterosexual married couples in India: challenges to the HIV prevention program. Health Edu Behav. 2004;31(1):101–17.

46. Mukhopadadhyay S, Nandi R, Nundy M, Sivaramayya J. Gender dimensions of HIV/AIDS: a community-based study in Delhi. New Delhi, India: Institute of Social Studies-Trust; 2000.
47. Nag M. Sexual behavior in India with risk of HIV/AIDS transmission. Health Transit Rev. 1995;5:293–305.
48. Bill & Melinda Gates Foundation. Avahan, the India AIDS initiative: The business of HIV prevention at Scale. The Bill & Melinda Gates Foundation, New Delhi, India; 2008.
49. Chandrasekaran P, Dallabetta G, Loo V, Mills S, Saidel T, Adhikary R, Alary M, Lowndes CM, Boily MC, Moore J, Avahan Evaluation Partners. Evaluation design for large scale HIV prevention programs: the case of Avahan, the India AIDS initiative. AIDS. 2008;22 (5):1–15.
50. Pandey A, Mishra RM, Sahu D, Benara SK, Sengupta U, Paranjape RS, Gautam A, Lenka SR, Adhikary R. Heading towards the safer highways: an assessment of the Avahan prevention programme among long distance truck drivers in India. BMC Public Health. 2011;11(6):15.

Open Access This chapter is licensed under the terms of the Creative Commons Attribution 4.0 International License (http://creativecommons.org/licenses/by/4.0/), which permits use, sharing, adaptation, distribution and reproduction in any medium or format, as long as you give appropriate credit to the original author(s) and the source, provide a link to the Creative Commons license and indicate if changes were made.

The images or other third party material in this chapter are included in the chapter's Creative Commons license, unless indicated otherwise in a credit line to the material. If material is not included in the chapter's Creative Commons license and your intended use is not permitted by statutory regulation or exceeds the permitted use, you will need to obtain permission directly from the copyright holder.

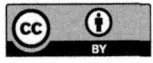

Chapter 6
The Way Forward

The field of self-care interventions is new, fast moving, and multi-disciplinary. There is a need to explore the way ahead in advancing the field so that self-care forms an integral part of health programs. In order to move this agenda forward, a comprehensive strategy is needed. This includes training health professionals on SRHR self-care interventions; providing education to potential clients; making self-care technologies available and accessible to potential users; promoting the use of digital and online resources to accelerate self-care; and providing research-based evidence for the formulation of policies and programs.

6.1 Training Health Professionals on SRHR Self-care Interventions

New approaches in training and education of healthcare providers are needed in order to institutionalize sensitive and effective use of self-care interventions. Healthcare providers include doctors, nurses, midwives, community health workers, and pharmacists, among others. Grassroots NGOs and community-based organizations (CBOs) are also important healthcare providers, especially for hard-to-reach communities.

It is important to revise curriculae of health professionals so that they are embedded in the principles of human rights, gender equality, increased user autonomy, and health literacy to empower and support confident decision-making. These training programs should focus on community-based curriculae with special emphasis on communication, compassion, and a person-centered approach to care; self-care interventions should be integrated into the curriculae for health professional education and training; training should be on holistic and integrated health care and sensitization to institutionalize empathetic attitudes which take into account the broader social, psychological, spiritual, and religious context of people's lives. Issues of power and vulnerability to support increased autonomy and empowerment should be addressed. And innovative research, technologies, digital and online resources, interactive learning, and other innovative forms of training should be integrated to reinforce comprehensive learning of information and practical skills [1].

Training curriculae for professional development should mandatorily incorporate knowledge and sensitization about vulnerable and marginalized populations, serving to break existing stigma and discrimination. Preparatory curriculae for healthcare professionals should be equipped with knowledge about new interventions and opportunities that will serve the needs of the potential users of self-care. Healthcare providers need to be provided with adequate educational and communication training to address sexual and reproductive health issues of the vulnerable and marginalized communities. Training programs should be designed to enable teacher–student and patient–physician communications address the importance of healthy and sustainable self-care practices.

6.2 Education of Potential Users on Self-care

It is critical that appropriate and effective educational programs for the public and potential users of self-care interventions are initiated and sustained. Education programs and community interventions through workshops, dialogue and other means should address sexually dominant notions, stigma, gender inequality, and the overall perceptions of gender and sexuality. These programs should pro-actively and regularly involve stakeholders, most importantly, policy-makers, and community representatives.

Mass media platforms should work toward censoring regressive attitudes towards sexuality, gender fluidity, and gender equality and should ensure appropriate portrayal of communities. Alongside academic education, mass media has the potential for addressing the traditional psychology of people by providing exposure to the third gender in society. These messages could be more effective if they are reinforced by known and famous personalities who serve as champions for the cause.

As a part of the school curriculum, age appropriate comprehensive sexuality education should be undertaken. Moral education and moral policing of girls should not be the "sex education" in schools; it should include gender-unbiased delivery of factual information. Information should be provided to adolescents on SRH, contraception, and STIs. There is a need to organize educational campaigns and programs for addressing issues related to STIs particularly HIV/AIDS. These campaigns should address the impediments to SRH such as HIV non-disclosure and criminalization of consensual sex in MSM, FSWs, and transgender.

6.3 Self-care Technologies

The following self-care technologies, including drugs, devices, and diagnostics, are currently available: oral contraceptives, emergency contraception, contraceptive patch, self-injectable long-acting contraceptives, diaphragm, abortion with misoprostol, self-testing for STIs, HIV self-testing, pre-exposure prophylaxis, and post-exposure prophylaxis (PrEP) [1].

There is a need to develop educational programs for the community to provide information about the availability of these technologies and where they can be accessed as well as on their indications and contra-indications, side-effects, and follow-up schedules. Factors including privacy and confidentiality, empowerment, convenience, and access are viewed as important by potential users of these self-care technologies [2].

6.4 Digital and Online Resources on Self-care

Digital health is creating opportunities and challenges around how information and services can be accessed and delivered. Alongside the trends in digital health, advancements in self-administered family planning methods, self-testing, and screening for sexually transmitted infections such as HIV and HPV and self-administered abortions are leading to a new paradigm of self-care interventions in the field of sexual and reproductive health and rights with particular implications for women [3].

Digital health enables self-care in several ways. The first is as a stand-alone self-care intervention, for example mobile apps for better home-based care and risk assessment during pregnancy. The second is using digital technology in combination with self-care commodities such as instructional videos for more effective use of HIV self-testing kits. Third, at a health systems level, digital health offers the opportunity for better continuity of care through the use of shared health records accessible to clients and health professionals.

The combination of digital health and self-care is accelerating the movement toward person-centered health and shifting the center of gravity for many health-related activities from a clinical setting to people at home or in their workplaces. This takes the notion of task shifting in health to a whole new level by enabling people to directly access and use commodities and services that have previously been entirely in the domain of health professionals or administered in a health facility. Mobile apps and online ordering services have become new intermediaries with Internet drug stores and pharmacies [4].

6.5 Research-Based Evidence for Policies and Programs

Research and analysis of self-care reported in this volume on men who have sex with men (MSM), transgender, female sex workers (FSWs), and long-distance truck drivers starkly underscores the serious paucity of research on these vulnerable and marginalized communities. There is a need to build on this research as well as to undertake research on other vulnerable, marginalized communities such as substance users, poor urban slum children and adolescents, poor rural women, migrants, and disabled persons. Research on these vulnerable communities would provide the evidence needed for the formulation of policies and the design of programs to address their multiple health, education, employment, and legal needs.

Self-care practices for vulnerable communities have special relevance as these communities remain unserved due to the serious barriers that they encounter in availing services from the formal health system. A major barrier is the stigma and discrimination that they face when accessing health care from formal healthcare providers from both the public and private healthcare systems. Research on their self-care perceptions, sources of information, barriers, motivations to practice self-care, and what they do when self-care fails would provide important insights for promoting self-care among these communities.

There is a clear need to systematically study self-care practices so that effective policies and programs can be formulated to address the needs of the general population as well as those of vulnerable and marginalized communities. As the design of these policies and programs has to be tailored to the needs of the communities they serve, it is critically important that research-based evidence on these communities is made available. Thus, it has been possible to design and scale-up self-care interventions for FSWs in several contexts because research to empower and mobilize this community provided insights for ensuring consistent condom use, thereby significantly reducing the incidence of HIV and other STIs in this community. Migrant FSWs are a specially vulnerable group for which interventions are not available because research-based evidence is needed to design and implement appropriate strategies.

Policy advocacy was employed over long years to legalize consensual sex among men. There is evidence that MSM are not a homogeneous group. There are several individual groups of MSM. For program strategies to be effective, they must be tailored to the needs of individual groups of MSM for which research-based evidence is required.

Self-care by consistent condom use by long-distance truck drivers, an important bridge population for the transmission of STIs/HIV, led to decreased prevalence of infection and its spread. This was an outcome of a program designed to make highways "safer." Safer highways meant increased exposure to HIV prevention interventions and consistent condom use by truckers with non-regular female sex partners.

Strong policy advocacy made it possible to acknowledge the legal rights of transgender. Policy advocacy undertaken jointly by NGOs, lawyers, researchers, and the community itself made it possible to convince policy-makers to recognize their special needs and to frame appropriate laws for the transgender community. These laws have enabled transgender to get voting rights and procure identity cards that specify their self-perceived sexual identity. In April 2014, the Supreme Court of India passed a landmark judgment reaffirming individuals' rights to choose their identity as male, female or third gender. This Supreme Court judgment in its verdict also instructed the central and state governments to develop inclusive social welfare schemes and ensure greater involvement of the transgender community in policy formulation.

However, accessing formal health and education services and employment opportunities remains difficult for the transgender community primarily because of the stigma and discrimination that they face in society. Thus, despite small wins, there remains a long road ahead to address the needs of marginalized and vulnerable communities. It is, therefore, important to prioritize research for obtaining the evidence for designing policies and programs. These efforts must be continued and sustained to promote sexual and reproductive health and rights and prevent HIV among vulnerable and marginalized communities.

A dynamic and flexible research environment driven by a collaborative ethos is required for undertaking future research. This research should include the contribution of the users of self-care.

Some of the elements of research undertaken in India may provide important leads for conducting research on marginalized and vulnerable communities in other countries. Future research must focus on the development and delivery of self-care interventions. The following are some research questions that need to be addressed: Is stigma and discrimination a driver for the use of self-care interventions within the healthcare system? Will a specific healthcare intervention improve coverage, reduce out-of-pocket expenditure, and be responsive to current and emergent population needs? Are health workers supportive or resistant to self-care interventions? Studies on self-care interventions for SRHR should advance knowledge on a holistic approach to health and well-being by reducing disparities and vulnerabilities and advancing universal health coverage (UHC).

To better understand the effects of self-care interventions in people's lives, implementation strategies need to be linked to clear outcomes. Successful mainstreaming of self-care interventions will therefore require monitoring and evaluation earlier on. While monitoring and evaluation is common practice for program implementation of focused health interventions such as the number of ante-natal visits for maternal health or use of anti-retrovirals for HIV treatment, it is far less common in domains where policies and programs are aimed at an organizational change. Introduction of quality self-care interventions is a true paradigm shift in the way health care is delivered. Its potential to bridge people and communities through primary health care to reach UHC is underexplored. Moving forward, researchers, policy-makers, and practitioners can consider the participant narratives regarding the need to consider both the heterogeneity of self-care interventions of SRHR and the needs and lived experiences of diverse populations. These lay persons' and healthcare providers' perspectives underscore the urgent needs to increase access, reduce stigma and discrimination, and improve knowledge for self-care SRHR interventions to increase UHC in order for individuals and communities to realize their SRHR and for countries to achieve the Global Development Goals [5].

References

1. World Health Organization. WHO self-care interventions for health: sexual and reproductive health and rights, global values, and preferences. A survey results. Geneva: World Health Organization; 2019.
2. World Health Organization. WHO consolidated guideline on self-care interventions for health: sexual and reproductive health and rights. Geneva: World Health Organization; 2019.
3. World Health Organization. WHO guidelines for digital health interventions. Geneva: World Health Organization; 2016.
4. Patricia M & Pierre M. Digital self-care must be approached by the health sector with eyes wide open. BMJ Suppl. 2019;29–30.
5. Narasimhan M, Logie CH, Gauntley A, Ponce de Leon RG, Gholbzouri K, Siegfried N, Abela H, Ouedraogo L. Self-care interventions for sexual and reproductive health and rights for advancing universal health coverage. Sex Reprod Health Matter. 2020;28(2):1778610.

Open Access This chapter is licensed under the terms of the Creative Commons Attribution 4.0 International License (http://creativecommons.org/licenses/by/4.0/), which permits use, sharing, adaptation, distribution and reproduction in any medium or format, as long as you give appropriate credit to the original author(s) and the source, provide a link to the Creative Commons license and indicate if changes were made.

The images or other third party material in this chapter are included in the chapter's Creative Commons license, unless indicated otherwise in a credit line to the material. If material is not included in the chapter's Creative Commons license and your intended use is not permitted by statutory regulation or exceeds the permitted use, you will need to obtain permission directly from the copyright holder.

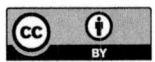

The manufacturer's authorised representative in the EU is Springer Nature Customer Service Centre GmbH, Europaplatz 3, 69115 Heidelberg, Germany. If you have any concerns regarding our products, please contact ProductSafety@springernature.com

Printed and bound by CPI Group (UK) Ltd, Croydon, CR0 4YY

25/03/2026

02078177-0010